An Optimist is Buried with a Wine Collection

A Journey through Stage IV Throat Cancer

by

Michael R. Carter

Edition 1.1

Copyright 2015 Michael R. Carter

*"Recommend to your children virtue;
that alone can make them happy, not gold."*

Ludwig Van Beethoven

This book is dedicated to my wonderful children, Sarah and David. May they seek out, capture, and defend the moral high ground.

Without Dr. Martinez and Dr. Jansen this book would be significantly shorter and written by someone else.

I owe so much to my wife, Laura, for many things including unwavering support and constant encouragement to never quit.

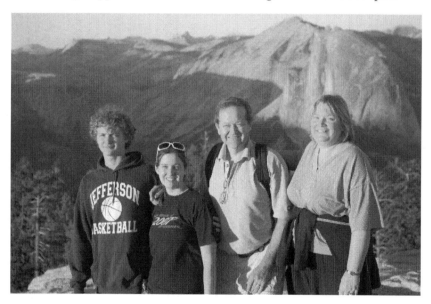

Foreword

By Sarah B. Carter

"Daddy, tell us a story!" Night after night I would call, tucked-in on the top bunk, Dave on the bunk below. Back then I couldn't get enough of Dad's stories. The ones about his friend, Al, and Sven the Duck (who was quite the family man, for a duck) were my favorites. Some of them I knew well enough I could tell them myself. I was a smart little kid. Dad loved this about me. He would teach me stories or punch lines to his favorite jokes, and get me to tell them with him to his friends.

Dad: "What do you get when you cross a blueberry with an elephant?"

5-year-old Sarah: "Blueberry elephant sine theta!"

Nothing is cuter than a 5-year-old telling trigonometry jokes.

Unlucky for Dad, this adorable phase of my life didn't last forever. I became a pre-teen and then a teenager. I was no longer asking for the stories every night. I had heard them all so many times already: Area 51, the police escort in New York City after 9/11, Madeira Hill… Granted the selection had expanded since I was five, but so had the opportunities for embarrassingly telling these stories to my friends.

If you know my dad, then you know the worst part was just how excruciatingly long some of these stories became. I swear, a 5-minute story turned into a 30-minute saga with an intermission for refreshments from the lobby! We all (Mom, Dave, and I) developed tactics for dealing with this, ranging from finishing the story ourselves (my go-to plan), leaving the room (Mom's favorite), or giving Dad "the fingers" (Dave's a pro).

Don't worry; "the fingers" were just like a peace sign, like your elementary school teacher would signal when she wanted to quiet the class. These fingers had a similar meaning, asking for quiet. They also meant, "Dad, this is the second time I've heard this." Or third, or fourth... you get the idea. Despite our best efforts, the rest of the audience would always be laughing by the end of the story, *encouraging* him! I guess my dad is funny?

Maybe my genes have predispositioned me to be immune to his humor. That must be it. I was genetically coded and the dad-humor immunity set in along with my pre-teen obsession with Justin Timberlake (correlation?).

Right around this same time, when I was in the 8th grade, still fresh from my first *NSYNC concert in the 7th grade, (I went with my teacher, how dorky was I?) Dad got sick. They shielded me from it for a while as best they could, but like I said, I was a smart kid. I knew what factorials were in the 3rd grade! (Thanks, Dad. Maybe that's why I saw my first concert with my teacher.) They couldn't hide it from me forever.

The first surgery took place while I was on a class trip to Washington, DC, before I knew I would be moving there a short year later. I called home five times that day, and got no answer. That was enough to panic a 14-year-old girl across the country from her family. But I kept my cool and enjoyed the rest of my trip. It turns out that was why they hadn't told me anything yet. They wanted me to have fun and not worry. Well, looking back, I'm glad they shielded me from some of the truth. In the words of Jack Nicholson, sometimes, "You can't handle the truth!" They told me a few weeks later that it was cancer, but what would teenage-me have done knowing the 20% survival rate? (I punched Dad in the arm when he told me that statistic a few years later.)

The truth is, though, I probably didn't need much shielding from Mom and Dad. I shielded myself plenty from what was going on. I have a few choice memories from this period of my life: filming the cool radiation treatment machine with my video camera (I was in my movie-director phase that summer), Dave racing toward Dad with the puke bucket and diving just in time, those awesome cookie baskets that Dad let us eat... But most of the rest is gone.

I don't even remember visiting the hospital post-surgery. I know it happened, but it's a blank for me, along with most of that year. I made myself busy with other things and dealt with stuff the way any teenage girl would, by NOT dealing with it. I refused to read the weekly updates, too. I was living it; I didn't need to read it!

But now, 10 years later, and 10 years smarter, and 10 years luckier to still have my dad, I am SO GLAD he wrote it all down. And SO GLAD he is a storyteller. I've outgrown some of my distaste for his stories (but not my love for J.T. – seriously, how does he still look so good?) and I think the stories in this book are probably going to be my favorites of all.

As I read these for the first time, I realized how brave my father was, and how genius. He kicked cancer's ass and he did it laughing the entire way (maybe no one else was laughing at his jokes, but you can always count on Dad to laugh at them for you). Humor got him through this, and his laugh is what we love best about him. I'm so proud of him, not just for beating cancer against the odds, but for writing this book and inspiring others to face life with a smile, no matter what it throws at you.

Mostly I am grateful. In years to come when I want to share these stories with my own kids (hypothetically, assuming my Dad didn't ruin my chances by teaching an 8-year-old girl factorials…) I will be able to grab this book. I'll be able to share the stories I heard as a kid, and the stories from my own childhood that shaped my family. They might not be exactly the truth – just warning you in advance – but they are *a truth*. And that's good enough for me.

So, Daddy, will you tell us a story?

Love, Sarah

Preface

"I unclosed my eyes."
- The Pit and the Pendulum, Edgar Allan Poe

"Don't worry, you won't remember a thing..." were the last words I remember as I lay on the table. I was rapidly approaching the event horizon, beyond which lies the unknown. I was supposed to count down from 100. Only the anesthesiologist and the three nurses know how far I got. I probably made it to about 97. Modern drugs are absolutely spectacular.

Then there is a giant blank in my life. So empty that I have no idea how long it was. It could have been five minutes, five hours, or five days. Something important was happening and, fortunately, I was completely oblivious. The future of my life, both its quality and duration, was in their hands. I hadn't known any of them two weeks ago. They did have my $250 co-pay, so I knew they would take me seriously. I had scribbled something on the consent form about "refundable if not successful." They had scratched that out. They intended to keep that $250 no matter how this turned out. This was not like a car repair where, if they don't fix the car you can take it back. This was the real deal.

Now it's just a big blank. This was the most important thing to happen to me since birth (with maybe a few exceptions) and it's just a black hole.

"What's happening? Where am I? Where's Laura?" I whispered to myself.

I unclosed my eyes and there she was. The first thing I saw as the first photons leaked between my eyelids was my wife of twenty-two years and ten months. She was my partner in life. She had been with me every step of the way since we had "fallen in love" at Indiana University in the shadow of the General – Robert Montgomery Knight. Bloomington, Indiana was a great place to go to school if you were a basketball fan or a music major. I was both.

Her first words (or at least the first ones I remember) were, "Hey! You made it."

I realized it was over... I had survived... for now...

"What did they do to my back?" I asked as I emerged from the drug-induced coma.

"You're ok." She replied. The tears were being pulled down from her eyes by gravitational forces. "I love you," she whispered as she gently held my hand.

I had survived. She was here. I was here. Wow! Life is good. I could feel that gentle, assuring grip on my hand, careful not to hit the IV. Her hand was shaking a bit but she was there with me. Why the tears? This had been a stressful week for both of us. There was much uncertainty about the path ahead (if there even was a path). Did she know something or was she just happy to see me? Don't ask... yet... First, be glad you're here to fight the next fight...

"My back! What the hell did they do to my back?" I asked again.

"You're ok. You made it. I love you." She whispered again.

"I love you too. Are Sarah and David OK?" I asked.

"They're fine. They're with Grandma." She replied softly.

"Can I see them?"

"I told them to wait until tomorrow to come visit." She said, knowing the kids might not be ready for this.

"How did it go?" I asked as if she might know.

"You made it... I love you." She reaffirmed.

"How long was I in there?"

"You made it... I love you." She reaffirmed again.

"How long?"

"Nine and a half hours… you made it." She said with her soft voice shaking a bit.

"That doesn't sound good. Did Dr. Jansen have lunch?" (I asked the important questions first.)

"You made it!" She reaffirmed for the n-th time.

"Did they get it?" I asked hoping she might already know and be willing to tell me.

"They don't know yet… I love you." She said quietly.

I had a feeling that she had talked to the doctor. She did know something. It wasn't good but I had in fact made it through this second surgery. Just ten days prior, they had removed a swollen lymph node from my neck and made an initial cancer diagnosis. The path ahead was uncertain but the prospects were not good. Terms like "unknown primary" and "partially differentiated squamous cell carcinoma" were being kicked around. I could only partially differentiate the terms but I was beginning to understand their meaning and get at least partially scared. Diagnoses that have terms like "partially" and "unknown" are not good. "Fully" and "known" might sound worse but they are not.

The "They don't know yet" response was not unexpected. They never want to tell you bad news in the recovery room. They probably don't know exactly what they got yet but they probably have a pretty damn good guess. It's not like they've never done this procedure before. They probably told Laura something and asked her to let me "recover from the anesthetic" and then they would tell me. Maybe that was the source of the tears, or maybe she just loved me and was happy to hold my hand. Yeah that was it. She was happy to hold my hand. This Dr. Jansen knows what he's doing. I have confidence in him (based on very little real data, just a gut feeling). Besides, what option did I have but to be confident in him? I had made it this far. I get to hold her hand. I get to see her tears. I get to complain about something new – my back.

An hour or so later, Dr. Jansen finally came by to see us. He had obviously talked to Laura, I could just tell from her words and body language. She hadn't said a word about it and I had backed off on the questioning – obviously getting nowhere. If there was bad news, maybe it was best if it came from him. I had a feeling that his nerd-like interpersonal skills would enable him to tell me. Surgeons like him need to have some emotional separation from their patients. They lose too many to develop close relationships. I'd much rather have a skilled surgeon in the operating room than a socially-skilled hack in the recovery room.

On the other hand, I had more than one goal. I wanted to survive. There was so much to live for. I had a driving sense of mission at work – make a difference in homeland security. I had two weddings to go to: Sarah's and David's. I had countless grandchildren to read to. I had intended to teach each of them pi to at least twenty significant figures before they went to kindergarten. That would serve them well in this dog-eat-nerd world. (You never know when you'll be stranded on a desert island and need to know pi (accurately) to survive.) There were people in my life that needed to know how much I cared for them. I had a wife to grow old with. I had bets on the table that I needed to win. I had always wanted to hike the John Muir trail, see the Pyramids of Giza, and enjoy the man-made wonders of Paris, London, Florence, Frankfort, and Lexington (the great cities of Kentucky). First things first: I had to develop a connection with this surgeon. I decided to cut to the chase.

I asked him a critical question he had never had to answer in the recovery room before: "What flavor today?" He had told me a few days before that he always took a can of Ensure into the operating room for long surgeries and would sip it for his lunch to keep his strength. I really didn't give a damn about the flavor but it drew a quick smile from the introverted-ultra-nerd-life-in-my-hands surgeon. This was progress toward one of my life goals (bringing a little humor to the nerds of the world).

"Vanilla." He snapped back, knowing exactly what I was asking about.

"I thought you preferred chocolate." I quipped as though this conversation was important. We both knew this was a diversionary tactic that I was good at. Humor and avoidance are great tactics to deflect emotions during stressful situations.

"Variety."

"Well… How did you do?" I asked, trying to actually cut to the chase.

"You made it." He said as if that was the most important thing at the moment.

My definition of "made it" likely went beyond his. I did have a pulse. I could still cast a shadow. I could convert CO_2 into O_2 [I must be a plant. I mean O_2 into CO_2]. I was still increasing the entropy in the universe. I was conserving both energy and angular momentum. Given half a chance, I think I could fog a mirror. My definition has a few more things in it than these, like: I want to be a threat. [This is not what it might sound like. It will become crystal clear in Chapter 16.]

"How soon can I play the piano?" (I love that old joke.) I continued before a response emerged from his puzzled face. "Did you get it?"

"Yeah" he said with a bit of confidence – how big "a bit" was hard to read.

"Margin?" I asked.

"We don't know yet." He replied showing how big his "bit of confidence" was.

That did not sound very good. I could see the tears reappearing in Laura's eyes. She knew something. Dr. Jansen had talked to her. I could sense it. This was not as good as they wanted me to believe. They had done this to my Dad. I was in the waiting room with my Mother when the surgeon told us that Dad was in the recovery room and the news was very bad. Stage IV pancreatic cancer is as bad as it gets. It was his death sentence. "Untreatable.

There is nothing we can do." It was everywhere. "We'll tell him in a few days... after he recovers from the surgery." Dad died in peace and with his dignity intact six weeks later. I knew he was going to die two days before he did and I just knew he could read it in my face.

Was this the tear in Laura's eye? Or was it allergies? Maybe there was dust in her contact lenses? Both eyes – yeah – that was it – it wasn't even a dusty day inside the hospital but two perfectly timed, well-placed dust particles would explain it all.

"I couldn't get as much as I wanted. The tumor was pushing up against the carotid artery. If I cut too deep then you wouldn't have made it out of surgery. I tried to cut out as much as I could. We'll have to wait until the pathology comes back to see if we got any margin" said Dr. Jansen.

I hate pathologists even though I don't know any. They only want to see you after you've lost the ability to talk back. I'll bet their medical school curriculum doesn't require Bedside Manner (BM-101). They are well trained at pulling you in and out of the cold, horizontal file cabinet. I wonder what they think when they hear something in their stethoscope (if they even have one).

I was bound and determined to fog that mirror, cast that shadow, increase the entropy in the universe, and read "Moo, Baa, La La La" to my yet-to-be-born grandchildren. My daughter Sarah could calculate factorials in the third grade. Her future children could beat that!

"By the way, what did you do to my back?" I asked Dr. Jansen.

"Nothing. Why?" He replied a bit puzzled.

"It's killing me." I exaggerated.

"It's probably just a pinched nerve from nine and a half hours on the table" he quipped.

Later that evening, my Mom and Brother, Ed, came to visit. They looked scared. They loved me. Mom cried. Ed joked a bit. We told some old stories. I was scaring them. They were scaring me. Maybe they had seen something that I hadn't seen yet (me) and I really didn't know how bad I looked. Maybe they knew something I didn't know.

This didn't really hit me until the next day when a close friend of mine, Joe Ronchetto, came to visit. Joe had retired from work a few years back and had undergone treatment for prostate cancer. It had scared us all but Joe had beaten it like a champ. Joe and I had worked together in the nuclear test program at Lawrence Livermore National Laboratory: me as a young "physic-er," he as an experienced "old-fart electronic-er." This is a natural rivalry. Joe had developed a nickname for me, "Peckerhead." In Joe's world, "PeckerHeaD" was short for PhD. He used my nickname often, loudly, and proudly. The situation never mattered. I was always "Peckerhead." Every day we would flip coins for a soda. The afternoon cry: "we match, you pay" would ring out in Trailer 1280 at Livermore and more often than random statistics would support, Joe would emerge the winner. "Old Fart Luck" it should have been called.

Joe came into the room uncharacteristically holding a small bundle of flowers. Joe Ronchetto with flowers? My world had changed. He took one look at me and turned as white as the blank pages of his engineering notebook. The handful of flowers wilted in his hands. I had yet to fog that mirror (or even see my image in it) but it was clear to me from the wilted bundle of daisies and the deer-in-the-headlights look on Joe's face that I looked like hell. He didn't call me "Peckerhead" that visit. He always called me "Peckerhead." Joe was nice. I get plenty of nice from everybody else. From Joe, I needed verbal abuse. Now I wasn't sure I was going to make it.

My two children, Sarah and David, did finally come to visit. Sarah was in the eighth grade. David was still in elementary school. They were too young to really understand what was going on. They knew Dad had cancer but they didn't know much more and they were probably afraid to ask. Seeing me on the hospital bed, looking like God-only-knows-what, didn't help them.

I cried when I saw them and thought about their wonderful lives ahead. There is nothing I wanted more in life than to watch them grow up into the absolutely wonderful people I know they will be. I'm sure my tears scared them. Or maybe not: They had seen me cry before. I always cry during The Parent Trap. Those poor twins were separated right after birth because their parents couldn't get along, only to be reunited at summer camp. What self-respecting modern man doesn't cry when Hayley Mills and her identical twin sister, Hayley Mills, pick up that guitar and sing, "Let's get together?" Identical twins look so much alike.

These tears were clearly different. I'd be home soon on the long road to recovery and I'd need my family as much as they needed me. They would be there for me. I knew I could count on that. The Grandkids could wait a few years. I hoped I would be there with them. Life was going to be good. The alternative was not an option.

Edgar Allan Poe had it right. He might not have known it but he was talking to us:

"I WAS sick - sick unto death with that long agony; and when they at length unbound me, and I was permitted to sit, I felt that my senses were leaving me. The sentence - the dread sentence of death - was the last of distinct accentuation which reached my ears."

Every cancer patient feels this way, and none of us can write like Edgar Alan Poe

As bad as this might be, I wanted to bring on the future. I had things I had to do. I had goals in life. I wanted to win as many Tour d' France races as Lance Armstrong. I was not ready to quit.

…Not even close...

Chapter 1

"Daddy, Tell Me a Story!"

"Ask me the questions Bridge Keeper. I am not afraid."
- Sir Lancelot, Monty Python and the Holy Grail

Every night, night after night, I would hear the call. The call was never ending, until I responded. I'm not sure how my kids learned to ask me for the thing I love most in life: telling stories. We had a few simple bedtime rules when our kids were little: no matter how late it was, they could always have a glass of milk and they could always get a bedtime story.

Everyone knows the phrase "It's not just a job it's an adventure" or "It's not the destination, it's the journey." Well, I think differently. It's not an adventure or a journey unless it results in a good story. The great thing about stories is that they are fun to tell, over and over and over again until one or more of the parties falls asleep or gets questioned about the details of the particular version of the story being told. Now, don't get me wrong. There is always only one correct version – the version being told! Others may remember incorrectly. Others may have misheard or misunderstood the "real" version. Truth, history, and facts cannot be allowed to get in the way of a great story. Nor should great stories ever be constrained by previous renditions or an uncertain remembrance of the "facts." This is, of course, the danger in actually writing them down. Someone may think the written version is the "correct" version. Never! Like it was for Orwell and Churchill, the pen of history is mine. But let us never be constrained by the written word.

Many of these stories are "famous" in our family. The great Alan Ropp became the source of many a story in my children's early years. Paul Alan Ropp was a friend and role model in high school. Al was two years ahead of me and was sort of my "hero figure." No one was ever more clever, exciting, or mysterious than Al. Al was a real genius – with all the inspiration and issues that came along with the genius ride. Al composed a violin concerto that was performed with full orchestra accompaniment at his high school graduation. Al graduated from Indiana University in two years with a degree from the school of music. He followed that by a year in England building harpsichords. Al was hit by a car at least three different times during his high school days. To be clear, that was at least three different times and at least two different cars. I looked up to him as a source of all that was fun and exciting. Monty Python, classical music, travel, adventure, risk, Indiana University; all these passions began with an "Al story."

There are also the other classics: The dead fish, my first date with Laura, the three month long trip to Siberia, my near death experience as a child on Madeira hill, Margaret's brownies, Area 51, my very close encounter of the fourth kind with Beth the lingerie model, our trip to Tule Lake in northern California, the rogue wave and snowball from God, and Sven the Duck. You name it and I could and have told a story about it. Have I bored the kids? Probably, but they kept asking for more. Has it bored me? Never!

As I embarked on a new journey, to recover from this nasty bout of head and neck cancer, I wanted to take the time to document the saga and get some of the old tales down on paper. In case I don't make it – someone else can tell the stories. In the more likely event that I actually do live forever, we can print it and I can read it to you. Or even more likely, I can just improvise.

This book is an attempt to record the accounts of the treatment and recovery process. Every Sunday night for the first six months or so, I wrote a letter and emailed it to my friends and colleagues. The intentions were many: to let my friends and colleagues know I was still alive, to keep them up to date, to provide an easy mechanism for them to write to me, and to keep my sense of humor and attitude as positive as possible. These letters are shown, in nearly their virgin state in *italics*. To put the letters in context (and provide some background on the story lines) I have added the account of how I got to the diagnosis and a few interspersed stories about myself, my family, and my closest friends. Also included are a few of the "Once upon a time" bedtime stories I told the kids when they were little.

Even though every cancer case is different, all patients share one thing: the need for support. Their support network needs support too. I assume that even the doctors need support. They sure act like it.

As hard as it may seem at times, there is one thing, and sometimes only one thing, that every cancer patient is in charge of: their attitude. There are times when depression dominates and your attitude does not seem within your control. There are times when the value of a positive attitude gets questioned. How can it possibly matter? I don't know exactly why, but I am convinced that, at a minimum, a positive attitude can't hurt. It certainly makes it easier on those around you. One cannot beat cancer with attitude alone. On the other hand, without hope and optimism, why even bother to fight?

Fight to win. Fight to fight another day. Fight to survive.

So, here we go! As Sir Winston Churchill said when asked if he was afraid of how history would view him, "History will look upon me fondly because, I will write it."

Have you ever noticed that really good stories often don't get started until about chapter seven?

Chapter 7

NEVER AGAIN!

"We're on a mission from God."
- Jake and Elwood Blues, The Blues Brothers

I remember exactly where I was on September 11th, 2001. We all do. Just like I remember exactly where I was when Lee Harvey Oswald was shot and killed. People as little as a few days older than me remember the Kennedy assassination. I was too young to remember that day in November of 1963 but just two days later I was a five-year-old sitting in my suburban Cincinnati living room watching Saturday morning cartoons on our black and white TV (without cable, a remote control, or TiVo) when my first lasting memory was made. I remember my Mom crying. Really crying. She had just seen someone shot and killed on live television. The nation and my Mother were already in shock and then – right in front of all of us – another killing. America would never be the same.

On September 11th I was in seat 4D on United Airlines Flight 222 from San Francisco to Washington Dulles. I was a scientist at Lawrence Livermore National Laboratory working on non-proliferation research & development projects. My classified documents were wrapped and sealed neatly in my briefcase under the seat in front of me. My seatback and tray table were in the full upright and locked position. My seat belt was buckled low and tight across my lap. My portable electronics were turned off until ten minutes into the flight. My emergency procedures card was recently read and returned to the seatback in front of me. The emergency lighting and exits had been identified, including the ones behind me. My carry on bag was safely stored in the overhead compartment poised and anxious to shift during flight. I tell this story like we're flying but the plane was still boarding, and we were still resting safely on the tarmac at SFO, gate 83.

Our research and development team had made some important contributions to our national security. We took pride in explaining these contributions in long PowerPoint presentations with convoluted, classified arguments, riddled with complex equations understood only by socially-inept audiences of the willing. We were doing some really good things – trust me. Little did we know, the world was about to change for the worse.

The pilot came on the intercom in a soft, confident voice – you know how those former military pilots are when they are flying a plane full of civilians: "Good morning ladies and gentlemen, we're in for a slight delay this morning. Air traffic control has asked us to hold here at the gate for a few minutes. I'll update you when I hear more from ATC in a few minutes. We don't expect a long delay. Thank you for choosing United Airlines."

Across the aisle from me in seat 4C, a man was talking on his cell phone – both the boarding door and the cockpit door were still open. He says to me, "I'm talking to my daughter. She's in New York City and she says a plane has just hit the World Trade Center." I'm thinking – "Some nut in a private plane. Stupid people. I'm on a mission to brief a critical, classified program to one of those three-letter Government agencies. One destined to search for and confirm the production of weapons of mass destruction in proliferant countries. Let's get this plane off the ground."

A few minutes later Mr. 4C whispers to me across the aisle. "There's been a second plane crash into the World Trade Center."

"That's odd." I thought out loud. "Another stupid person? No way!"

About that time, two foreign men get up from first class and exit the plane. The pilot comes over the intercom and announces that we're going to close the boarding door but we'll be sitting here for a bit longer. "We don't expect a long delay from Air Traffic Control." No explanation, just more delay. Has he heard about the plane crashes? Now we're trapped. My classified documents are still safely sealed and stored in my briefcase – my hand carry authorization card tucked in my wallet. I'll feel funny taking my briefcase to the airplane restroom so, I need to go easy on the liquids. Luckily, we don't have to wear handcuffs and cuff the briefcase to our wrist.

Mr. 4C is still talking to his daughter on his cell phone. She apparently is in a skyscraper in midtown Manhattan with a view of the twin towers out her window. "Oh my, she says one of the towers just fell."

"That's impossible! She's crazy!" (I'm not sure if I said this out loud but I sure thought it.)

Now I'm thinking: I need to get off this plane and back to work to store these documents. We're not going anywhere anytime soon. I find myself sitting in the comfortable confines of seat 4D. Seat back and tray table in the full upright and locked positions and I don't have a clue. No clue as to what's going on outside this 757. No clue as to what to do. I knew the 1993 attack in the parking garage of the World Trade Center was masterminded by an Islamic fundamentalist cleric in New Jersey. There was a connection to al-Qaeda but to me, all these fundamentalists groups were the same: all driven to take the world backwards. They were intent on fighting the long war against progress. Technical progress, social progress, and religious progress (if there is such a thing) were all a threat. Having failed to knock down the symbols of progress in 1993, maybe they were intent on striking again. And now some crazy lady on a cell phone in New York is telling us that they have succeeded? Seems unlikely.

After an hour or so, the pilot reopened the boarding door and encouraged us all to either stay on board or stay in the boarding area. We expect an update from Air Traffic Control within the hour. I have no idea what to do but I'm thinking, "I'm going home." If this plane ever does get off the ground, it's going without me and my documents.

The first quest though was to find a TV. SFO? No chance. It's a great airport but – on 9/11 it was TV free.

On the drive home, KCBS-740 was covering the story full time – interrupted "on the 8s" with traffic updates from around the bay area. By the end of the day, their traffic reports would compete with WKRP's Les Nessman – both without their fleet of helicopters and fixed wing aircraft. Without a visual confirmation, I still had a real sense of disbelief. It was just not possible to knock down either tower of the WTC – and certainly not both. It just can't be true. Early talk about terrorism filled the airwaves. There were more hijacked planes. One had crashed into Camp David. One had hit the Pentagon. One had crashed at the State Department. Others were being shot down by the military. The White House was being evacuated? What the hell was going on?

Arriving at work, I made a beeline to my conference room and turned on CNN. Now more than three hours after the attack began, the visuals were being replayed over and over again. I guess it was true. I guess I had to believe. Talk about Osama Bin Laden was becoming widespread. Other than check on my wife and kids, I had no idea what to do. That "good idea" would take a week to come. In the meantime, I'd just go through some motions pretending to do something. In reality, I was like much of the rest of the nation – in shock. How could we let something like this happen? Why wasn't President Bush doing something?

About two weeks later, we finally got the phone call. Could we fly our cameras over the WTC site? Could we deploy our cameras invented to find the bad guys overseas to understand the disaster site in lower Manhattan? You bet we could. Finally! We're on a mission from God! Time to turn my career to Homeland Security.

It took a few months for this all to set in but finally, sitting alone on the red picnic table in my Mother's basement over Christmas vacation in 2001, I hacked out an email to my boss telling him I was interested in an assignment in Washington. In particular, there had been a call for personnel to help staff the new Office of Homeland Security under former Governor Tom Ridge in the White House. I had decided to try to get my name in the hat. The lab system works in strange ways. My name was removed from said "hat" because they had "more senior names" they were pushing into the hat. They were pushing a list of more experienced management types (Division leaders, former Division leaders, ex-

Division leaders, disgruntled Division leaders, formerly disgruntled Division leaders, Division leaders emeritus, disgruntled Division leaders emeritus at large.) You know these kinds of guys. I wanted to be considered at least in the "future disgruntled Division leader category." I had a future. I could do "future disgruntled."

The list was built (without my name), placed into "the hat" and submitted to the Washington decision makers. Similar "hats" from Los Alamos and Sandia National Labs were filled and sent to Washington for consideration. As the story goes, "the hat" was returned to the lab with many of the names scratched out and my name written in (as I like to say – "in crayon"). (The crayon writing process is a special access program so don't expect to uncover the source of the crayon sharpener. Some stories are better left untold.)

I finally interviewed for the job with Dr. Penrose Albright in May of 2002 (the government moves kind of slowly). I knew they were writing the President's Homeland Security Strategy but I did not know they were in the process of writing the President's plan for the new Department of Homeland Security. The administration had repeatedly stated that they did NOT need such a department but they were also working under the leadership of Richard Falkenrath to craft their own strategy for a Department of Homeland Security. I thought I was interviewing for a position at the Office of Science and Technology Policy (OSTP). OSTP is the office led at the time by Dr. Jack Marburger, the President's Science Advisor. I had known Dr. Albright (from here out known as "Parney") from previous days working for DARPA and he apparently knew of me. We got along great from the get go. Parney had a vision for the "not yet announced Department." In particular, we were in charge of developing and implementing the vision for a prime role for Science and Technology in countering the threats of Weapons of Mass Destruction (Chemical, Biological, Radiological, and Nuclear terrorism – CBRN).

I wanted the job! Whatever it was.

A few weeks later, they announced the proposed creation of the Department of Homeland Security. After messing around most of the summer trying to get a start date, I finally showed up in mid-August. August is a nice time of year in the former swamp land of Washington, DC. I was there at 8am on day-one of the Transition Planning Office. I parked myself right outside Parney's door and got ready to do the transition planning thing... whatever that was going to be. Joining Parney was Dr. Maureen McCarthy. Maureen was the Chief Scientist from the Department of Energy (actually the National Nuclear Security Administration (NNSA)).

It was one of the most exciting times of my life. We were in "White House" office space just a few blocks from the real White House. We were in the real White House every week. We were right there – responsible for the biggest overhaul of the Federal government since the creation of the Department of Defense after the Second World War. To beat that, the Science and Technology Directorate was being formed from whole cloth – by about ten of us. In the world of pioneers and settlers, I was a pioneer. I would eventually learn the frustrations of being a pioneer in a world of settlers but that was going to be a while. You know what they say, "you build it and the settlers will come." Well, we were building it and they were coming.

We developed a close-knit team led by Parney and Maureen. I was working radiological and nuclear counterterrorism. John Vitko worked bio-security. Greg Suski concentrated on information and analysis. Bill Lyerley worked medical countermeasures. John Cummins focused on infrastructure protection. Holly Dockery concentrated on standards and international programs. Mike Mitchell worked business practices and Charity Azadian kept us on task. Our primary focus was Chemical, Biological, Radiological, and Nuclear terrorism prevention. We were in the business of investing in science and technology to prevent the use of weapons of mass destruction. This was no easy task given current state of the countermeasures and the consequences of such events. We had a lot to do. There would be many unknown obstacles ahead: governmental and personal. Bring them on.

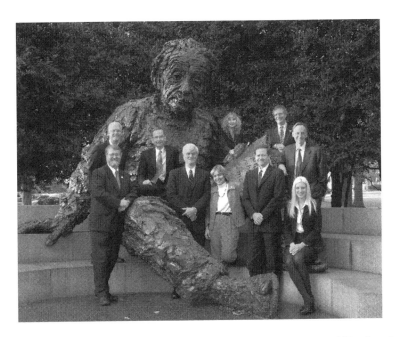

The Department of Homeland Security Science and Technology Transition Planning Office team. Left to right: Bill Lyerly, John Cummins, Dr. John Vitko, Dr. Parney Albright, Dr. Maureen McCarthy, Holly Dockery, Dr. Mike Carter, Mike Mitchell, Greg Suski and Charity Azadian. Dr. Albert Einstein sitting quietly in the background.

Chapter 8

"Pathetic"

"A woman is the only thing I am afraid of that I know will not hurt me."
- Abraham Lincoln

The cancer journey started during our Christmas vacation in 2002. Our family was traveling to the Midwest, as we always do, experiencing the joys and struggles of cold weather and extended family visits. Laura's parents live in Plainfield, Indiana, just outside Indianapolis. My Mother lives in Cincinnati. Our visit to Cincinnati, like every year, would include the annual quest for Skyline Chili, Graeter's Ice Cream, and Montgomery Inn (the Rib King). The Rib King is the home of the BEST pork ribs in the world (Bob Hope's favorite until the day before his death). There is no better ice cream in the world than Graeter's ice cream. It's Oprah's favorite and in this case, Oprah is right – there is no better ice cream anywhere – not in State College, PA – not anywhere. Skyline Chili is my favorite. There is nothing like it – it's not "real chili." Cincinnati Chili is unique and really good. Try it twice and you will agree. (Implicit in that last statement is: try it once and you might not.)

This year would present a new complexity beyond attempting to break the record for the most number of Skyline trips per day or, the most consecutive days with a Skyline run or, the quickest consumption of a pint of Graeter's Black Raspberry Chip ice cream. This year would include all those challenges and more. I had decided to get Laura a real gift this year. I had decided on a rock! A face-center cubic carbon crystal was just the thing every woman needed. I had scored a beautiful diamond "engagement" ring to celebrate our 21st and 1/2 wedding anniversary. This was a gift that would finally answer the mail and clear all my previous transgressions. You know – 21&1/2 is a big one – 43 is the carbon half-year. Getting up the nerve to actually give it to her is the longer story. It was nearly documented in the annual Darwin Awards. It nearly made "America's Funniest Home Videos." You can find the short version on Wikipedia under "loser." I nearly got voted off the island. Suffice it to say, I was *nearly* a threat.

I had a great autumn that year away from home saving the free world from al-Qaeda and the other bad guys. I must have been developing a bit of a guilt complex. I decided I needed to get Laura that long-neglected diamond ring. I worked with my friend Holly Dockery a fellow Transition Planning Office detailee from Sandia National Laboratory in Albuquerque and famed jewelry reseller. We had scored a really nice diamond.

Giving the ring to my wife, Laura, was the next step. Sounds easy? Only if you don't know Laura.

There is something about my wife that intimidates me. For those of you who know us both – you may find that hard to believe. For those that know us well, you know exactly what I mean. I have a long track record of botching the whole gift thing. Year after year of Valentine's Day massacres, anniversaries to not remember, birthdays and Christmas gifts that will only be mentioned in future court proceedings. Oh the humanity! But I told myself this was going to be different. Finally, I had gotten her a gift to remember. I was intent on doing it right, making it special. Just once in my life, this was a chance to shine. Get it right! Now I needed to step up to the challenge, but I had to define "right."

The advice started to pour in, especially from the women around the office. "Don't blow it." "It needs to be romantic." "It's personal – don't put it under the tree." "Don't try to be funny – don't put it in a box, in a box, in a box." Well, there went my first ten ideas. I finally decided I'd take her out to dinner before Christmas – just the two of us – and give it to her then. We both like food. We like food a lot. Skyline Chili might not be the right venue. To us, life revolves around food. Food is very romantic. I had a plan. I just needed to get the ring to Indianapolis and meet up with her and the kids. I could do this, except, as the saying goes, "Shit happens to nice people, too."

On the last night in DC before the holiday, Holly finally gave me the ring. All I had to do was store it safely one night and then get myself and the ring on the plane to Indiana. I had a great idea. I'd lock it up overnight, nice and tight, in my office desk at the White House instead of carrying it back and forth to my hotel. As I walked into the room I realized I had not put the desk drawer key on my key ring but instead had just dropped it in my pocket of my $1,299 Hickey Freeman, state-of-the-art, off-the-rack, Nordstrom's-men-store suit. Well, since that day, Hickey and I have had a difference of opinion about the genuinely crappy quality of their pocket material and the subsequent key-falling-down-the-pant-leg phenomenon. I now had a $6,000 ring, locked in a White House desk and a hole in a $1,299 suit (plus alterations, tax and tip) – and no key. This was going to ruin my plan. MY PLAN! MY GOOD PLAN! MY ONLY PLAN!

Panic set in the next morning when I asked Cindy Christian, the lead office administrator, to mobilize the White House Locks and Keys Task Force (WHLKTF) and get my lock open. Normally, this was a two-week process and yet it had to happen before my afternoon flight. Cindy suggested I get the key number from the lock to facilitate her attempts to accelerate the WHLKTF process. Thankfully, there was some good news in all this. It turns out that every drawer in the office area was keyed with the same lock. I mean every drawer in every cube on the entire floor. One key. And since the furniture was new, every drawer still had a key in its lock – except for one – the drawer with my wife's diamond ring in it. Sometimes the key gods are kind. Exactly how they had planned to "lock things up" in the White House was not clear... but I was a winner!

Ring in hand, I met Laura and the kids in Indianapolis. Life was good. I was back on plan. We spent the evening with Laura's family in the quiet suburban town just west of the airport. We woke the next morning to the familiar sound of the massive fleet of FedEx planes taking off from the Indianapolis airport just a few miles to the east. They were busy this time of year, delivering last minute packages in what I like to think of as the pre-staging logistics before Santa's visit. We packed up the car, ring in pocket, and headed for Cincinnati. It was our normal drill. We had two weeks, two cities, and two families to visit. Life was good. I had a plan (sort of).

Well, before I knew it, it was Christmas Eve. And I realized, my plan was not really that good. In reality, I was chickening out. I thought I'd give it to her on Christmas Eve night in some private, romantic moment. Romantic? Private moment? Christmas Eve in Cincinnati? Christmas Eve was that annual, predictable panic where she yells at me for procrastinating as we wrap the last presents. By "we" I mean, I sloppily try to wrap them and she rewraps the ones she cares about because my tape or paper folds or whatever is just not good enough. The kids are just going to rip the paper to shreds first thing in the morning – who cares how neatly the paper is folded? Does Mrs. Claus second-guess Santa loading the sled every year? We put out cookies and milk (the kids were a bit old for this but I can't tell her that), talk about the stockings and our inability to get 4 "good ones that match" (like guys care about such things)… Yeah…I care! (or I can fake caring if really necessary.)

The next thing I knew, we were loading the kids' stockings with skittles and dental floss, drinking the milk, eating the cookies and heading for bed – with the ring box still in my pocket. Romantic would just have to wait. Christmas Eve is only romantic in the movies. I needed a plan. I had a plan. I had a "new" plan. Maybe I could do the box in a box in a box plan in the morning.

In reality, it was clear that I had no plan. I was chickening out again. I was trying to listen to the great advice of all my friends so I decided not to wrap it and put it under the tree. I'd give it to her Christmas evening. That was it. The moment needed to be special. Romantic. Something we'd remember. A story we could tell our Grandkids. Or at least, a story we could tell ourselves because the Grandkids really don't care about such boring Grandma and Grandpa stories. (He reminds himself as he types – who will read this anyhow?)

We were joined that Christmas by Aunt Sara (my Mother's sister) and Uncle Don. Uncle Don had given Aunt Sara an awesome diamond ring under that same tree a few years ago. He had wrapped it in a box, in a box, in a box (the outer box with a brick in it). Uncle Don was cool. The ring was awesome. The look on Aunt Sara's face was very memorable. Maybe I should look for that brick. Nah... We finished opening Christmas presents, ate dinner and packed up the car to head back to Indianapolis. Christmas evening was the new plan. Wait! Christmas evening? That wouldn't work. Not at her Mom and Dad's house. Give it to her in front of her family? Not a good plan.

The next thing you know, I'm planning another romantic dinner out on the town for the 27th of December. This would be perfect: just the two of us. This will be romantic. Ruth's Chris Steak House in downtown Indianapolis. That's Ruth'ssss Chrissss Sssteak Housssse – I can hear the USDA Prime rib eye steak sizzling in boiling hot butter on a 1,400 degrees Fahrenheit plate (that's only about 500 degrees Kelvin) – on what turned out to be a cold, windy, miserable, dangerous, snowy evening – canceled! We do not go out in the snow unless we have to. We did "have to" but she didn't know it.

Well, New Year's Eve is always nice and romantic (except at the in-laws'). It began with a fight over returning the nearly-spectacular gifts I had carefully chosen for her to Coldwater Creek in cold, windy, snowy, nasty weather. It ended with us switching channels to see the last seven seconds of the ball drop. Switching from? Some old synchronized swimming movie from the 1940's starring Ethyl Merman or someone equally as uninteresting. I bet you didn't know Ethyl Murman was a synchronized swimmer. Well – she isn't. It was Esther Williams (who can't even sing) but that's not the point. At 12:00:02 it was back to the backstroke. Ethyl/Esther was hot in that 1940's swim suit. I was the only one drinking that evening. I was drinking for cause.

Next thing I know, I'm watching New Year's Day bowl games with that damn ring still in my pocket. This was not going well. But I had a plan. I really only had one plan: "Continue to re-plan." As they say at work, "it's not the plan, it's the planning." Well, It was not the planning either. It was just a mess... Maybe it's the fear... Fear of failure and fear of success both rolled into one.

January 2 – that was the night. I got another reservation at Ruth'sss Chrisss Sssteak Houssse (Did I mention the USDA Prime Steaks sizzling in butter? Life was gonna be good!). It was cold and windy with a chance of snow and we almost canceled twice but I finally got Laura in the car. I had a plan: we'll order champagne and I'll give it to her with a toast (a toast I haven't thought through but – I'm a good winger – I'll wing a toast!). Well, she passed on the Champagne. We don't even like Champagne. Plan? Caesar Salad didn't seem like the right time (not sure why). We like Caesar Salad and Ruth'sss Chrisssss has a good one (not as good as Wente Restaurant in Livermore but – we were not at Wente – if we were, I'd spring with the damn ring right then!)

Next to us was a famous football player from the Indianapolis Colts (we didn't know who he was but – he was very famous in his own mind and the mind of the hot babe with whom he was sharing his wealth.) To him – this would be a "small ring" I'm sure. Little did he know he was eating at the table next to a famous physicist from the soon-to-be-Department of Homeland Security. He too, famous in his own mind, with his own hot babe (soon to have said "small ring" – if I can figure a way to give it to her).

The next thing I know, we were finishing off two of the best steaks on the planet and having a great time. I felt very brave. It was time to order the Molten Chocolate Cake (her favorite) and cough up the damn ring. Well, Laura didn't want desert – she wanted to go home to her Mom's chocolate cake with caramel icing (her real favorite). I order the damn molten chocolate cake anyway (with two spoons) and we shared it very, very slowly– it was very, very good and very, very romantic – now was the time. It was nearing perfection. It does not get better than this. I felt brave. Just do it!

The next thing I know, the bill is paid, we were putting on our coats, hitting the restroom and heading out the door – the ring still in my pocket… I was really on a roll. Downhill. We emerged from heaven and ventured back into the cold. Back into the dark. Back into fear. What is my problem? Why am I so damn bad at this? That damn molten chocolate cake with two spoons was the perfect time.

Well, it was cold and windy and cold and windy and it was a two-block walk to the car (parked on the square in downtown Indianapolis). The Christmas lights were still up on the square (it is Indiana, they may never take the Christmas lights down from the square – I don't know) and it was a beautiful sight (until we get in the car – get it fogged up and slowly warming). I finally decided – this is the time. We were shivering in the dark, in the car, in the cold, in the car... and I finally cough up the ring... In the dark, in the car, in the cold, in the dark. It was special... I'm really good a this... it was a De Beers moment. I think she likes it. This should have been my plan all along. This is the stuff they reject for De Beers' commercials it's so good. This is the real world. Diamonds glimmer in the light. Diamonds shiver in the dark.

There are two versions to the end of this story: Laura's and the truth. She claims to have said, "It's beautiful." (Did I mention how dark and cold it was?) I recall she said just two simple words "you're pathetic." I'll leave the judgment to the reader. We have no official transcript but I know what I heard. I think both versions capture the moment. Both versions were true – It was beautiful and I am pathetic.

She finally knew why I'd been acting so strangely over a shared piece of molten chocolate cake.

The homemade chocolate cake with caramel icing was very good that night (as it always is). Little did I know, it might be my last.

The next morning, January 3, 2003, while proudly shaving in front of the bathroom mirror at my in-laws house, proud to no longer have a beautiful diamond ring box protruding from my pocket, I noticed a swollen gland under my right chin.

No pain. No fever. No fear.

Just a "little lump."

Chapter 9

It's Just a Swollen Gland

"Very strange people, physicists – in my experience the ones who aren't dead are in some way very ill."
- Mr. Standish, "The Long Dark Tea-Time Of The Soul"
 - Douglas Adams

Just like all swollen glands, it was nothing to worry about – probably an infection – no pain, no blood, no guts, and no fever. It would go down in a few days. After a grand and glorious vacation with multiple trips to Skyline, a very successful gifting experience, and multiple pints of Black Raspberry Chip ice cream, I went back to Washington, DC to save the free world. Laura and the kids returned to California. I let the little lump in the neck go for about a week with no noticeable change (and no pain) and finally decided to go to the local Kaiser hospital on Pennsylvania Ave in DC (just a half dozen blocks west of the White House). Just like all Kaiser visits, it starts by getting a medical record number (a one-day process for a visitor to the east coast) and a $10 co-pay. I saw a nurse practitioner, Ms. Casa. She started me on some inexpensive antibiotics but also referred me to the Ear, Nose and Throat department immediately. I thought nothing of it except the inconvenience of coming back the next day.

I arranged for an appointment with Dr. Maria "Tess" Martinez (Ear, Nose and Throat surgeon) the following afternoon and started the antibiotics given to me by Ms. Casa. At this point, this Doctor stuff was like stopping and asking for directions – men don't like it (especially while women are watching) but sometimes, you should just do it. The problem is determining if this sometime is significant or just another in a long train of "I'm okays."

Dr. Tess Martinez was absolutely fantastic. We took an instant liking to each other (or at least me to her). She inspected me (my first throat scoping) and said I likely had just a clogged salivary duct. The throat scoping was special: they spray some cocaine-like substance in your nasal cavity and run a fiber-optic light up your nose and down your throat to look around. (It's worse than it sounds but after a few dozen times, you get used to it). She immediately started me on a stronger antibiotic (one of those $300 ones that you get when the cheap stuff doesn't work and the HMO is afraid you might sue them). But the cheap stuff had not failed to work yet. That should have been a sign but I was just following directions. Hey – at least I was stopping to ask. She told me to come back in two weeks.

Two weeks passed and I could notice no change. I also had no other symptoms that I associated with the lump in my neck. In hind sight, I had been experiencing a few "symptoms" like: increased snoring, sleep apnea and acid reflux that were all apparently associated with the as-yet-undiscovered obstructed airway. A friend in DC recalls that I complained of a slightly sore throat during this time but it must have not been too bad – I don't remember it. I probably complained about a few other things too but I don't remember any of them either. Life was just too good in the White House. We were making Big Government. This was the biggest Government reform since the establishment of the Department of Defense in 1947. Who needs a War Department? A Department of Defense is so much better.

Dr. Martinez decided to put me on another cycle of even stronger (and more expensive) antibiotics to reduce their legal liability. (I mean, see if the "infection" would respond.) At this point she was still saying she suspecting a clogged salivary duct. Again "come back in two weeks." I should have gotten the hint. $800 of antibiotics for a "clogged salivary duct" was a sign. She made me feel better by telling me she could feel the clog in my mouth under the tongue. She knows what she's doing. She's seen this before. She's a professional. She was almost certainly thinking something else but not talking yet. I still liked her a lot.

Two more weeks passed – it's now mid-February. I returned to Dr. Martinez, empty antibiotics bottle in hand, gland still swollen. At this point she must have been beginning to wonder. She still gave me the "clogged salivary duct" speech and ordered up an urgent (but not-life-threatening-urgent) CAT scan. Well, the CAT scan place was in Fairfax and I was car-free in DC – yeah, I know, I could rent one or take a cab but what a hassle. I put it on the "simmer" burner. I called and got an appointment but a "more important" work thing came up. I can't even remember what that "more important" thing was. I probably had to empty Parney's trash.

At this point, the CAT scan was threatening to get in the way of my annual ski trip with Ralph Haller and Ron Ewing to Crested Butte, Colorado. God knows how important skiing and male bonding is! The ski trip won! The male bonding was good! We drank some great wine, ate some red deer, elk, and buffalo, left the seat up, did some forearm bashing, made fun of guys who stop for directions, and talked about old "Pig Eye" (a story I can't tell because Laura might actually read this section and I would lose more than I would gain by talking). Pig Eye's fundamental theory of life is in fact true, but all males are sworn to secrecy. Life was great. Maybe not double-black-diamond-slopes-great but very, very good.

Now it's March and my friends and family are starting to bug me about getting that CAT scan done. It never pays to get family and friends involved in medical issues – especially ones you are trying to just wish away. Hey – IT'S A CLOGGED SALIVARY DUCT! Dr. Martinez told me so!

Finally, after another conversation with Dr. Martinez where she requested that I "get the damn CAT scan and get an extra copy of the film and DRIVE it to the office after the appointment" (saving a whopping two days). I finally called for a real appointment. At this point I'm still thinking it's just a clogged salivary duct. After all, she can even feel a stone in the duct with her finger (and I bought that story too). She's just trying to confirm her diagnosis and then start a treatment course to break up the clog. Sounds like passing a kidney stone through your mouth. Odd but I can do that.

The CAT scan day arrives but first I'm off to the FBI lab in Quantico. We're building a nuclear forensics program for DHS and FBI that will be second to none. This will be important someday, maybe even *really* important. So will my CAT scan but work always comes first. Well – once I finally made it to the radiation clinic, the CAT scan was fun. A little iodine in the veins and twenty minutes in the tube sounded like a big deal at the time and the pictures were really cool. (They don't tell you that the radiation dose is about the same as a person standing about 2.5 km away from an atomic bomb blast.) By the time I got the scan done, hung around for a copy of the films and got back downtown, Dr. Martinez's office was closed. Not having a better option, I took the films to work for amateur analysis.

Like all scientists we just couldn't wait for the real doctors so we studied the film and pulled a diagnosis out of our ass. We held the film up against the window of the office overlooking the Washington Monument, Jefferson Memorial and Reagan airport. If you looked to the right, behind the buildings and through the trees you could add the Lincoln Memorial to the list of national icons used as the film backlight. What a great job I had. What a great journey I was just about to embark on and I didn't even know it. Let me tell you – it's really easy to find an "expert" in Homeland Security to read your CAT scan. There were about ten of us rendering diagnosis and at least twice that number of opinions. The standard comments emerged from the guy from HHS – "Hey – your head's not hollow" or the Coast Guard "Damn! You're ugly on the inside too!" We had more diagnoses than we had MDs and PhDs.

One of the real Doctors (maybe the only "real Doctor") from our biodefense program, Dr. Mike Asher, walked by, saw the CAT scan film up on the window, took a quick glance and put his finger on the "anomaly" (obvious only to him) and said loudly "this person's going to die!"

Ouch… I thought, as the room quickly fell silent.

"Whoops, sorry. Whose films are these?" he asked, realizing that he had not done so well in his remedial Bedside Manner 101 class. Backtracking quickly, Dr. Asher said, "This could be anything. I'm only an epidemiologist."

I always point out there are at least two kinds of doctors. As the classic New Yorker cartoon of the maître d' on the phone taking reservations at a fancy restaurant asks, "Is that a medical doctor or merely a Ph.D.?"

Mike Asher was a medical doctor. Although he was just an epidemiologist – not an Ear Nose and Throat specialist or a radiologist or a pathologist or an expert in whatever I might have or not have. I still had hope. What the hell does an epidemiologist know about non-contagious diseases? Maybe he had gotten a B in CAT-Scan Reading in medical school. And a physicist should know more about CAT scans, and image reconstruction than any damn epidemiologist.

The next day was quite memorable. I had an appointment with Dr. Martinez at 2 pm and was planning a late afternoon train ride to New York City with Dr. Huban Gowadia to visit Brookhaven National Laboratory on Long Island. I was nervous but in "justifiable denial" given the "Whoops, sorry" comment from the epidemiologist and self-proclaimed "expert" from the night before. Huban and I ate lunch at a fine, hole-in-the-wall Thai restaurant on Pennsylvania Avenue near George Washington University (right near Kaiser's clinic in DC). Then Huban and I parted, destined to join up in a few hours and head to Union Station for the Acela train ride to the Big Apple. The trip was located safely in denial corner.

Dr. Martinez welcomed me and immediately focused on reading the film in my clutches (see image below). She took one look (about five seconds) and called for her scheduler. She requested a surgery slot ASAP. She needed to go in and get a biopsy. Surgeons love to get you in surgery. I think that's what they do for a living, hence the title "surgeon." This is an early indicator of how the medical profession works. If your city is sick, talk to the epidemiologist. If you have an ear-nose and throat problem, talk to the ear-nose and throat specialist. If you really want to find out why you died, talk to the pathologist.

The swollen lymph node was about the size of a chicken egg. "It's too big to be an infection," Dr. Martinez tells me. She also noticed an asymmetry in the tonsils and was planning a simultaneous lymph node biopsy and tonsillectomy with the corresponding two-week recovery time required for adults who get their tonsils removed. She reserved a surgery slot for the following Monday afternoon. Expect about a 3-4 hour surgery. Wow – that was quick. It's supposed to be harder than that to schedule surgery. Out for two weeks? Recovery? Didn't she realize I was working for Parney Albright? Dr. Penrose C. Albright! (OK, Parney is merely a Ph.D.) I can't believe she had never heard of him. This was not on track. And what about my trip to Brookhaven? Control of my life was shifting from one set of Doctors to another. The two communities are not known for their collaboration. I was caught in the middle. Parney was losing.

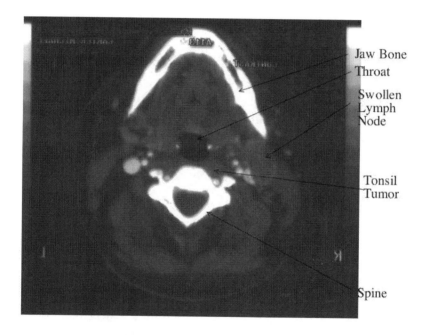

At about this point, I realize that this might be serious. Are four-hour surgery slots reserved in five minutes? I asked her, "What do you think this is?"

Her response was, "I don't know what it is."

I said, "I know you don't KNOW what it is, but what do you THINK it is?"

Then she said it. "I think it is Lymphoma."

"Isn't that a C word?"

The denial phase was almost over… The trip to Brookhaven was canceled… My life was about to change, right before my eyes.

After a bit of reflection and a very difficult call to Laura on the walk back to the office, I realized that I really needed to get home. Get home to California. Get home to my wife and kids. Home is where your wife is. Laura can put some popsicles in the freezer for me. Surgery in DC was one thing. A two-week recovery away from home was another. Little did I know how long the process was really going to take. Two weeks seemed like such a long time to be gone. I should be so lucky.

It's now April 2. I picked up a White House phone and called Kaiser Permanente in California. If they had caller ID they would pick up the 202-456-xxxx extension and know I was important. I don't think they had caller ID. The call started with some small bickering about "who did this diagnosis?", "where are you?", and "you need a referral to see a specialist – you need to start with your primary physician." I was finally able to get an appointment in the head and neck department for the following Monday (the same day the surgery was scheduled in DC). I could work the rest of the week in DC and head to California on Friday evening – denial is so sweet. I sat and thought for a while, torn between the two Doctor worlds, trying to weigh my near-term and long-term options. I called Kaiser back. Monday wasn't soon enough. I talked them into an appointment the next day. I called United Airlines. I want to go home! I've got to go home. There's no place like home. I need my wife.

I had dinner that night with a dear friend, Bill Kendall from Los Angeles. We broke into a great bottle of wine (my last for quite a while) and I told him how confident I was that all would be OK. I also told him I was scared. I didn't admit that to many people. I didn't feel scared very often. Bill was one of my role models with class, charm, character and smarts. I had told Laura about the artwork in his office in West LA. Describing the "kissing fish sculpture" on his coffee table in his office overlooking Santa Monica bay or the "mating elephant" artwork on the wall didn't really sell to Laura as "class" but – it really was. Laura, having never seen it, was not a believer based on my description alone. Someday, I'll get her to Bill's office and convince her.

I had run the Bay to Breakers race across San Francisco with Bill the previous year. Bill "ran" it with his heart monitor to be sure his heart rate stayed low. I "ran" it trying not to touch any of the naked guys. Not too many guys Bill's age still work everyday running a small company and making real intellectual contributions. I wanted to follow people like Bill. Following would have to wait a bit. The route I was on was not littered with leaders. I had no idea where I was headed.

After dinner I returned to my desk at 1800 G Street. It was late and I was alone in the office, but the last thing I wanted to do was go back to my hotel room by myself and get caught up in the denial, depression or anger cycles. That would have to wait. I had work to do (the denial phase). I was going to be gone for at least two weeks (denial). I'll just sit, work, and enjoy the view of the National Mall (denial). One last time (depression)? Finally, about midnight, I retraced the steps where I had lost my desk key only a few months before, this time carrying my CAT scan films. I would spend one last night in my hotel at DuPont Circle. This time when I checked out, I'd take my bags home to California (depression). It was time to get on with it (acceptance). Anger would just have to wait… In fact, I think I'll try to skip anger completely. (Hope!).

Chapter 10

Back Home in California

"Unfortunately, the immutable laws of physics contradict the whole premise of your account... That is one magic lugie."
- Jerry Seinfeld

I found myself back in California with my CAT scan films in hand. I met Dr. Cornelius Jansen. One quick look at me and my CAT scan film and he too realized we needed to go in for a biopsy. The "C word?" We were "going in" early the next week – as soon as we could get an operating room slot.

Surgery was scheduled for Tuesday the 7th (eventually postponed to the following day – Wednesday, April 8 – because someone was sicker than me? That was hard to believe.) Dr. Jansen is an Ear, Nose and Throat surgeon and is about my age. He trained at Johns Hopkins Medical School, practiced for ten years in Hawaii, and moved to Kaiser to work more with the patients than the insurance companies. I could buy that. He was your classic nerd but so am I. I really liked him. He was a real Doctor, not merely a Ph.D. He had a nice diploma on the wall. I needed him. I had better be nice. He had better be good.

I also started working on second opinions. The first order of the day was to get a solid diagnosis. I started talking with my sister-in-law's brother-in-law (Dr. Tim Miley) in Minneapolis. Tim is a pathologist and he began by giving me some questions to ask of my doctors. One important question for the surgeon before the first surgery was "why are we taking the tonsil? Isn't the key to the diagnosis the biopsy of the lymph nodes?" I asked that question in the operating room between countdown numbers 98 and 97 (just before the anesthetic took effect) and Dr. Jansen decided to only get the lymph node this first time in. I got to about number 96 and – the world just went away. They dug in and ran some cold sections of the inflamed lymph node in the operating room. The preliminary diagnosis was in: "Poorly differentiated, squamous cell carcinoma – unknown primary." It sure was nice to have a pathologist in the operating room with you – serving two functions – diagnosing the fresh tissue and standing guard in case he was really needed.

Recovery from this first surgery was a piece of cake (compared to what was ahead). So far it was just a small incision (about two inches) under the right chin and a full extraction of the chicken-egg-sized submandibular gland. A few good narcotics and a few days later, I was back at work. The medical system was off doing the formal pathology thing (finalizing the diagnosis) and also scheduling a second surgery. This next time would not be as easy. Assuming the initial diagnosis held (which it would) they were going for the full-up tonsillectomy and the highly-coveted "radical neck dissection" where they remove the sternocleidomastoid muscle, the lymph nodes and the jugular veins from the right side of the neck. They also started to talk about the longer treatment path – it did not sound fun... The two-week recovery was sounding better and better. The path ahead was going to be much longer (I hoped).

In the meantime, I wanted to make sure the diagnosis was right. Getting a second opinion was like... well... getting a second opinion. The system is not set up to help you do this. Kaiser first offered a second opinion from a physician in the office right next door to Dr. Jansen. I wouldn't need any additional tests. I wouldn't have to carry my files – they could just pull them up on the computer. It's easy. In my opinion, That was NOT a second opinion. It was more like a first opinion a second time.

They then offered me an appointment with a head and neck surgeon at Kaiser in Oakland. Again advertising that I wouldn't need any additional tests done and I wouldn't have to take my files. They could just call my file up on the computer. Well, this was a little better but still fell well outside my definition of a "second opinion." I didn't necessarily want more tests done but I did want an opinion from an "independent, qualified expert" (the best I could find). To me, this was not going to be another physician that might be limited in some way by the Kaiser system. Not that I felt there was something fundamentally wrong with the system, but an independent second opinion was important to me. With my life at stake, I really wanted to know exactly what I might die from. I wanted the tumor slides to go to Tim Miley and I wanted the patient to go to Stanford.

The system was also not set up for you to help them or help yourself. I had to fight the system almost every step of the way. Judy Kammeraad (a friend from work, about five years ahead of me on the cancer survivor timeline) had told me, "Remember, you are in charge of your treatment." But it was hard to be the Commander in Chief with no army and no training. Judy was in trouble herself. She had accepted the task of covering for me in DC for the two weeks (or more) that I was expected to be away. She was begging for a second opinion too.

One thing I had to do was to get slides sent to another pathologist (in this case Tim). The first challenge was to find the pathology department at the Kaiser hospital in Walnut Creek. I walked up to the reception desk staffed by those expert volunteers. I asked what I thought was a relatively simple question - "Where is the Pathology Department?"

"The what?" asked the volunteer behind the desk.

"Pathology." I replied thinking she might have just not heard me.

"I have no idea – not on my chart." (I thought, "Don't the volunteers walk around? Am I the first patient, living or dead, that ever asked to visit the pathology department?")

Well, it turns out the pathology department was about ten feet from the reception area in the "other hallway to nowhere." Unlike most other departments at the hospital, the Pathology Department sign was not meant to be read by living patients. I thought I was still alive so, not being sure of the protocol, I knocked on the locked door. I waited. I knocked again. I waited. I knocked louder.

Someone inside opened the door (just a crack) and asked, "What do you want?"

"I need to see a pathologist." I replied in my best "living" voice.

"Our pathologist doesn't see patients." (I thought – "at least while they are alive.")

"Please?" I tried. (Note to the researchers in the Library of Congress: sometimes the desperate patient's version of the event and the "actual" event captured on the security cameras differ just a little bit).

I finally got in and explained my situation to the people behind door #2. The pathology staffer (not the doctor) listened and agreed to send a set of slides to Minneapolis if I signed the right forms. Forms? Were signatures required from their "other" patients too?

The pathology slides finally made their way to Tim in Minneapolis. Tim looked at them and also forwarded them to the Mayo Clinic where one of the world's experts on the pathology of squamous cell cancers took a look. They must have experts in lots of things we have never heard of. I was glad there's an expert in whatever I have. There were a few "important" issues like – was this poorly differentiated or undifferentiated? Was there any indicator that might lead to the origin? This "unknown origin" thing was a bit scary. How could a tumor the size of a chicken egg (medium, grade A, organic, free range) come from an unknown location? These cancer cells' growth and distribution processes were just not clear to me (or the doctors). In any case, the diagnosis was confirmed by Kaiser's pathology, UCSF, the Mayo Clinic and Tim. Further surgery (the tonsillectomy and the radical neck dissection) was in order and I was officially sick – with the "C-word."

I was a Stage IV cancer patient and didn't really have a clue. The language was foreign to me: "partially differentiated," "squamous cell," "unknown primary," "Stage IV."

This did not sound very good...

... and it was not.

But I have something very important working in my favor...

Chapter 11

Lucky

"Carter, you're the luckiest guy I've ever met!"
- John Scarafiotti

"John, you need to get out more."
- Mike Carter

The second surgery on April 18th was not very pretty. It began just like the first with some small differences. They scheduled an all-day operating room. They gave me priority parking on far side of the fifth floor of the beloved parking garage. There was a $250 co-pay instead of the $50 co-pay for surgery number one. I need to reread that insurance policy. Lying on the gurney, I was told by the anesthesiologist that they were planning to "rigid scope" me again just like two weeks ago. They would again have me awake for that "stick a rigid scope down my throat" thing. I told her that they didn't do one the last time. She corrected me and told me about those "you forget everything we did to you" drugs. Wow! Good stuff. They have to keep you awake for the procedure but it's so bad, they have to make you forget it. I will nominate the inventor of that drug for the Nobel Prize in Medicine and Peace. Apparently, without him/her, this section would be significantly less funny. Life without anesthesiologists would be so much more memorable – but not better.

Nine and a half hours later, I was out. Dr. Jansen described the surgery as "the tonsillectomy from hell." There was very little margin (if any) between the tumor behind the tonsil and the carotid artery. I've heard of that "carotid artery" although maybe just as a spelling bee word. I think it's important. Add to that a four-hour radical neck dissection (it's worse than it sounds). I came out (alive) and I looked like hell. I hear if you die from the neck dissection surgery, they don't let you into hell because they're afraid you'll scare the other patrons.

I woke up and was in terrible pain. What did they do to me? They must have pinched a nerve in my back with me on my side for 9 &

1/2 hours. Just give me more morphine drip! The good news – they got margin. The bad news - maybe not as much margin as they wanted. It turns out that the Doctors are trained to NOT give you the straight story right after surgery (especially if the news is not good). They have this idea that "false hope" is part of the cure. I swear he mentioned margin with some sign of a smile. Maybe he was laughing at me. Maybe it was the drugs.

In the operating room they had taken a quick look at the tissues they removed from my neck and they didn't see any big tumors in the thirty-nine lymph nodes they yanked from my neck. The lymph nodes were gone along with two jugular veins and the Sternocleidomastoid muscle or some other complicated name for a muscle you can see, and the nerve feeding the neck, shoulder and whatever else. It was time to send the extracted tissue and lymph nodes off to pathology for a real look. The jugulars were now gone from the right side of my neck and fifty-two metal staples were holding me together (barely). How exactly the blood drains from the brain with one of the the jugulars gone is beyond me. They say it just drains down the other side. Does it really work this way? I have no idea but my back hurts so badly that I can't think about the neck thing right now.

Look in the mirror? – That was not a good idea. Thank God I can't get up. Thank God I have the back pain. It gives me something to worry about. It's apparently not pretty. Not pretty at all.

One of my best friends in life, Joe Ronchetto, stopped by the hospital at a particularly inopportune time – like – I was not looking good. I could tell by the look on his face that he was really scared. I could see the fear in the people around me. FEAR! Real Fear! Luckily, getting up to look in the mirror was not an option yet and I was not really sure how bad I looked. I just kept thinking, "I'm going to make it." I might be scared and deformed for life but I'm alive (at least for now). This wasn't about being attractive for the babes – this was about the pulse. Without the pulse, the babes don't matter much.

At this point, I began to work on more "opinions." I'm a big fan of second opinions.

Yeah, yeah I know the joke – real funny – "I asked the Doctor for a second opinion and she said, 'you're ugly too.'"

At this point, I really am ugly… but… I'm alive and I think I'll get better.

Chapter 12

The Weekly Updates

"I skate to where the puck is going to be."
- Wayne Gretzky – the Great One!

I finally made it home – miserable but surrounded by the familiar confines of the first floor of my two-story home. I also had the added benefits of cards, flowers and cookie baskets from fearful friends and family around the country. The path ahead was unclear except – there would be no cookie eating for the foreseeable future. For those of you inexperienced in the joys of throat surgery, sending cookies to a throat surgery patient is like sending a chair to Bobby Knight – he wants the chair – he knows what to do with the chair - but the chair in his hands just causes trouble. Send ice cream next time. Bobby likes ice cream. I like ice cream. Everyone likes ice cream… Graeter's Black Raspberry Chip would be good.

I was in desperate need of a coping mechanism. Hibernation? Panic? Anger? All possible. My kids know all too well that when I'm stressed, I tell jokes, I laugh, I smile. I'm listening and I'm taking them seriously but – I try not to yell and scream – I don't get mad – I joke (or try to joke). Consistent with my normal stress management mechanisms, I settled on a series of weekly email "updates" to be sent to my 250 closest friends. They would be brief and "informative" but that was only part of the reason for writing them. The updates served several important purposes:

They kept my friends and family up to date on a very regular basis. It even gave them something to look forward to – as odd as this might seem.

These emails helped to "break the ice" with my friends and family, enabling them to write back to me. People are often afraid and don't know what to say to a cancer patient. The patient is scared too. I wanted and needed to keep in touch with my friends and family.

They served as my coping mechanism encouraging me to look for the humor in the most dire of circumstances. No one wants to read a doom and gloom email even if the situation might be doom and gloom.

In hindsight, the mental battles ahead were every bit as important as the physical challenges. You hear stories about the power of positive thought in battling through an illness – the "mind over matter" thing. I don't claim that any of that is true. I do think the opposite is true – a negative attitude can do much harm. The struggle to maintain a positive outlook in the face of the unknown is not easy. These weekly updates were one of the keys to my mental mindset.

The updates also served as a mechanism to get informed on the path ahead. Even something as obscure as squamous cell cancer has been experienced by others… maybe not others on my direct distribution list but each of the recipients knows other people too. In this network are experiences and expertise, successes and failures, victory and defeat. Some of the opinions scared me. I was warned of skin rashes, "sun burn", dry mouth, weight loss, feeding tubes, and killer hiccups (whoo… I'm scared). These notes also connected me with other physicians with real experience.

The overall prognosis was not very good. I define "overall prognosis" as probability of survival. This is equal to one minus the probability of death. The 20% survival rate was not good but it was 20%. By the way – do the math – the probability of death was about 80%. Even though this number is larger, I'll talk about the probability of survival. I'd beaten odds worst than that before but for much lower stakes. I was told of many side effects: I would lose my sense of taste. I would lose my ability to swallow. I would lose my salivary glands. I was warned that I might never eat again. They talked of a lifetime on a feeding tube. One doctor told me; "For some, it is just too much trouble to eat." "Trouble to eat?" It's a joy in life. It's in second place on my list of favorite things (see my upcoming short story "Things men enjoy other than the obvious.")

A feeding tube? – I don't think so. Little did I know at this point how important that damn feeding tube would become. All the warnings were good and bad. One would think that being well-informed would be a good thing. It's not that clear-cut. Being well-informed can be very scary and depressing. "Well-informed" must be better than "poorly informed" but only if managed well. Well-informed seems like a must if a treatment path is to be chosen. It must be a prerequisite. Or – just trust the Doctors. I'm a Doctor but – merely a Ph.D. – not very helpful. You just don't know what lies ahead. That's part of the struggle. You just DON'T KNOW.

The right path ahead was just not clear to anyone. The doctors had seen people through worse than this. And, they had lost others in better shape than me. There is a reason they call it "practicing" medicine. They should practice on someone else and use those lessons to treat me. No – they are always practicing: even on me. There was more than one path? The paths ahead are scary and uncertain. What seems certain is that one path is scarier than the other, but it's more certain. I think I'll choose uncertainty. Everyone says your attitude matters but they really don't know or can't explain why. I'm not sure why attitude is important but I must assume it is, so, I'll have attitude and fight to maintain it. The alternatives - bad attitude and no attitude - don't seem right. The question is, can I keep it?

In the interest of my medical privacy, I reproduce the letters as they were – unchanged by hindsight (as tempting as that is). I only change the font. The original versions are shown in *italics*. I'll interlace comments and older stories (some connected to the cancer journey – some not) between the letters. The updates started just after my second surgery with a "letter" to my secretary, Tencia Leon (and my 249 other closest friends), expressing some concerns about the recent "trip" she had booked me on… I hope you enjoy them as much as I did.

At times, this was all I was enjoying.

Chapter 13

Dear Tencia

"What is our aim? I can answer with one word: Victory - victory at all costs, victory in spite of all terror, victory however long and hard the road may be; for without victory there is no survival."
                                    - Sir Winston Churchill

Dear Tencia

I have some concerns about my last trip. You booked me at the Kaiser Inn in Walnut Creek, California. Apparently, on April 18th I had an all-day meeting with a Dr. Jansen. The details of the meeting are a little fuzzy but it must have gone well because I ended up very hoarse (a good sign - I got to talk a lot I presume) and my neck is very sore (I guess I did a lot of looking around). The business part of the meeting went well. I do have a few complaints about the accommodations.

1) I think you forgot to give them my frequent flyer number so, when I registered in the lobby (they made me prepay) I used my United Visa card. I believe I got the frequent flyer miles for this. Next time - see if the Kaiser Inn has a frequent stayer program. I do think I got two free weekend nights. (I only paid for the first night - they called it a "co-pay" but I never met the other co.)

2) I prefer a limo to and from - riding with my wife is not only stressful but I am accustomed to a sort of "style" that doesn't include a wife and a mini-van.

3) If you could send me with a mask and latex gloves the next time I'd look less conspicuous. They have odd uniforms but I can adapt.

4) In the future, please request a private room. I thought our travel policy permitted this but with the struggles with the University of California management contract this might have changed. In the event that private rooms are no longer acceptable, please request an "other sex" roommate.

5) Try to get me in a room with a door that closes and locks. The maid and room service personnel, while friendly enough, were in and out of the room all night checking to be sure I was sleeping. I was, except when they were checking on me. Please request that the Inn issue them flashlights to avoid turning the room lights on in the middle of the night.

6) The food! I expect better. Normally I am permitted to eat outside the hotel. On this trip, they had me hooked up to some of the furniture and in a nightgown that was not appropriate for the local Ruth's Chris Steak House so, I ate from the room service menu. Their selections were very limited. They should be encouraged to expand their menu beyond the Jell-O, apple juice, and chicken broth selections. A nice filet or live Maine Lobster would have been nice.

7) The entertainment - please try to get HBO for me next time. I just don't understand why the lab picks such places for us to stay - Is HBO too much to ask for? - I need my fix! I did get to see some of the other patrons - we all seemed to have the same issues with the in-room robes - they really should wrap all the way around the backside.

8) The drugs were good - limited selection but they seemed to get the job done.

9) Please check for me - why did I have to give them blood to check out? Marriott does not do this (yet).

Thanks for the consideration on the above issues. This trip was not one of my finest. I really do expect to travel better. In the future, you could avoid all the complaining by just booking me in a Marriott – they seem to do a better job letting you sleep if nothing else.

Thanks for the support,

Mike

Chapter 14

Lupe

"Badges? We don't need no stinkin' badges!"
- Everybody who has ever worn a badge

Laura stayed overnight the first night at the hospital with me. My brother, Ed, (two years younger than me with a severely receding hairline compared to mine) had flown in from Minnesota to help. Ed decided to stay with me the second and third nights. My claim is that there is no better brother in the world than Ed. I would stack him up against anyone this side of Mother Theresa's brother Phil. He might even take Mother Theresa herself in a best of seven series. It might help if it were a "best brother" competition. She'd kick his butt in a "best mother" brawl. Ed's only vulnerability is ping-pong where history shows he has lost quite badly to his clearly superiorly skilled, and slightly older brother.

Ed was a major help as I was recovering from the surgery and the pinched nerve. I was absolutely miserable (and finally knew how bad I looked after making the mistake of glancing in the mirror in the bathroom). I scared myself. My good looks were at risk here. How was I gonna get the girls? With my math skills?

Ed described this phase of his life as the "wipe my brother's butt crack phase." Not so good for him but not bad for me. I promised to bring this up during our next ping-pong match as my score approaches 21 and he hovers in the single digits. As we approached midnight on the third night, the nurse's aid, Guadalupe, came in to check on me. "Lupe," as her nametag read, had been on duty the night before and had been very nice to us. She looked at Ed trying to sleep in a terribly uncomfortable chair and took pity on the poor guy. She said she would go find Ed a better chair. Ed and I went for a walk and when we returned, Lupe had found a big leather recliner in the doctor's lounge. She had placed the chair on a bed sheet and dragged it down the hall and into the room and placed it by the bed. When we returned, the chair just looked too comfortable to pass up (I was not sleeping well fully reclined in the bed) so I told Ed, I was sleeping in the chair. (Ed ended up sleeping the night in the hospital bed.)

When Lupe returned, Ed was out getting me some tea and I was resting comfortably in the new recliner. Lupe looked at me in shock and said, "Oh, Mr. Carter, I got that chair for your son."

"Son?" I must have looked *really* bad.

Extraction from the hospital finally came after night three. Dr. Jansen wanted to keep me another night but the comfort of the hospital was not enough. I begged for the exit criteria (must have a BM, hold down Jell-O, etc…) and proceeded to work the checklist hard. I needed to get home where I thought comfort was waiting.

They kept asking me, "On a scale from one to ten, how bad is your pain?"

"Zero" I said.

"Now Mr. Carter, it can't be zero." They replied knowing I was lying.

"Zero!" I insisted. "I want to go home." I repeated.

At one point they asked me if my morphine button was broken because they were not seeing the "button pushes" they expected. I told them, I'd rather go home than push that damn button. Get me out of here! I'm sorry if I diminish the need for morphine – the miracle drug. Morphine is good stuff to be sure but its use is on the exit criteria check list. I'm just one BM away from walking out of this place. It turns out they don't let you "walk out." They make someone wheel you out in a wheel chair. Must be a liability issue. I wanted to make a point and walk out.

Actually, I just wanted to go home! Wheel, walk, run, fly, or drive, I did not care. A Star Trek transporter would have been nice. Dorothy was right - "There's no place like home."

Chapter 15

The Recovery Begins

"As God as my witness, I thought turkeys could fly."
- Arthur Carlson, WKRP Station Manager

April 24, 2003

I thought I'd take a few minutes and update the "family" on how poor Laura is doing nursing her poor, helpless (yet still good looking) husband back to health. First - I plan to milk this for all the sympathy votes from Laura that I can get. That ain't easy!

I hope this "news" doesn't reach any of you off guard. My surgery was last Friday – 9&1/2 hours removing the right tonsil and a tumor behind that tonsil (surgeon called it the "mother of all tonsillectomies" (although I think he spelled it correctly)). The doctors think this is likely the primary but pathology will render its opinion sometime in the next few days. That was the first four hours. They followed this with what the experts in bedside manner call a "radical neck dissection." They must have learned this from the frog dissection days (although frogs make it through this better than people do). This process removes the lymph nodes from the neck along with one of those muscles whose name ends in an -oid plus the jugular veins and a few "non-important nerves." They work around the "important nerves" like the one that controls the heart rate and the breathing.

The recovery from this includes - learning not to complain about weird nerve signals, learning to drink Ensure, learning how to swallow a one cubic millimeter boulder in your mouth and learning how to sleep in a chair.

Last night was the best night sleeping to date. I'm still struggling with a very dry mouth and the nasal passages are still "congested." The combined mouth breathing, poor saliva production, sore throat and lack of morphine lead to about a two-hour limit on sleep in any one segment. I got about 3, two-hour segments in last night and another 2, one-hour stints.

My mouth and throat are still sore - eating is now officially on the WBS (sorry for the acronym to the family) - it means - it's really important and can't be considered a background or level of effort activity anymore. My fifty or so staples come out on Tuesday of next week. Until then, I am under strict orders to avoid metal detectors. I expect to start the radiation treatments sometime in the middle of May. They will likely push to combine with chemotherapy for an improved prognosis - we'll wait and see. We're working for a second opinion from Stanford (even before the first is out). I think we need some options and need to be better educated.

There is some good news - my brother, mother, wife and kids have been absolutely fantastic. Without them, I'm not sure this would be doable - with them, it's just a bad tasting piece of cake. The support from my friends and family has been overwhelming. My family doesn't even know about our FY 2004 budget line in the Presidents budget to Congress and they seem to like me. My kids know what their budget line looks like and they know their Dad is a soft target right now.

I'm feeling better and better every day - just not big enough daily changes to be "feeling better." Better get back to the harder task of resting. Thanks for everything,

Love, Mike

P.S. Today is my Mom's birthday and guess what - I don't even have a card for her. Are there any ideas out there?

Chapter 16

I am a Threat!

"Three things tell a man: his eyes, his friends and his favorite quotes."
- Albert Einstein

A few years back I found myself stuck in the Phoenix airport on my way back to the Bay Area from Houston, Texas. I had taken Continental Airlines to Phoenix and they had arranged to transfer me to America Worst Airlines (Sorry – America West) to expedite my return to San Francisco. I hate America Worst. Anyhow, the flight was late, I was tired and as they started to board, I realized I did not have a boarding pass, just a ticket. I went to the counter, the guy laughed at me and started to do that typing thing they do behind the counter. You know, the one where they have to hit 543 keystrokes just to see if they have any seats remaining on the flight boarding right in front of them.

He said, "Mr. Carter, there is good news and bad news. I have one seat left. It's a center seat in the back row and it doesn't recline."

"I'll take it!" I said (duh).

I accepted my fate and hopped on board. I snuggled into my beloved back-row, non-reclining, center seat realizing this would be a flight from hell – but what did I expect from America Worst? Dear God – Give me United Airlines!!!

A few minutes later, I looked up and an absolutely beautiful, redheaded, young woman was walking down the aisle toward the rear of the plane. My brain kicked in (or at least I think it's the brain): "Come on back baby. Come to papa. Right here baby. There's an open seat right here. Come on, make my day!" Sure enough – bang – the window seat – right next to me – maybe this flight wouldn't be so bad after all. Who cares about a reclining seat anyway?

Just after takeoff, I started up a casual conversation with her. You know: "So, heading home?" "Where you headed?" "Where you from?" "What do you do for a living?" JACKPOT! She was a model flying to San Francisco for a photo shoot. SUPER JACKPOT! Not just a model - she was a lingerie model. She went on to tell me her life story. Her dog, her husband, her house in Dallas, and her breasts were all beautiful.

She just happened to have her photo portfolio with her. She broke it out and began to show me some of the finer points of lingerie modeling. She explained that she didn't model for Victoria Secret but for the Mervyns' and JCPenneys' of the world. She told they loved her "red hair, all American looks, and perky, natural breasts." I glanced (slowly) in her direction and commented that her breasts did indeed look "perky and natural." This was going well. I'm not sure when the plane actually took off, but I did notice the flight was going very quickly. Why can't America Worst blow a schedule like normal? The conversation never veered far from her breasts (they were pretty special and we both seemed to be enjoying them).

It turned out, she had never met a physicist and she was "very impressed." This was perfect. I could tell her about quantum mechanics… and relativity… or we could talk about her breasts. This was not as easy as it may sound. And I didn't even have my physics portfolio with me.

Near the end of the fastest flight ever, she asked me how to get to her hotel in San Francisco. What did I know about getting around in San Francisco? I was getting a rental car and heading for home. I had my shot – I could have offered to take her to her hotel or, stay married and pass my next polygraph. I chose poorly. I told her where to get a cab or pick up the hotel shuttle or whatever – I forget. Married – I still am. Polygraph – here I come.

Her photo shoot was expected out in the Mervyn's insert of the Sunday paper in about a month – July 25th as I recall (not that I'm a numbers person but even all these years later, I still celebrate the last Sunday in July as Perky Natural Breast Day). That Sunday (July 25th), I was back in Houston and received a pager message from my always good-natured wife. It read, "They're natural and they are perky!"

I, of course, told this story to my friends at the weekly Friday Night Dinner (FND) get together at the Clower household. The universal question that emerged from everyone was, "Why do women talk to you about this kind of stuff?" The consensus opinion led by the ever-threatened Ellen Tarwater-Clower was (and continues to be) – "Mike, you're just not a threat."

That's not fair! I wanna be a threat!

Chapter 17

All You Can Eat

"No Soup for You!"
- Yev Kassem, The Soup Nazi, Seinfeld

April 28, 2003

Only two days until payday!

I'm feeling much better since the last update. If I keep improving at this rate, I've got a shot at becoming Pope when the slot opens up. Finally swallowing without labor and pain. I have developed a new and proven weight loss diet. Key points:

Eat all you want.

Eat whenever you want - I was averaging ten meals a day.

Add sugar to everything you want.

Consider popsicles a palette cleanser.

Eat wherever you want.

There is only one catch - The doctor will remove your "want." I call it the modified Suski diet. In Greg Suski's case he had Dr. McCarthy. I had a Dr. Jansen.

I lost 15 pounds in a little less than three weeks eating absolutely everything I wanted (and more).

Well - my want is coming back. Last night we had spaghetti with meat sauce. My helping could have been described as Calista Flockhart sized but - It was good. This morning it's oatmeal, bacon, and eggs. I'm gonna gain that weight back (or at least some of it).

I went for a couple of walks this weekend. It was one of those beautiful spring weekends in California where we can only say the weather is not worse than rest of the nation (normally we can say confidently that the weather is better). Calling what I did a "walk" might be a stretch. More like a stroll - the pace of the Easter Parade from the old movie with the funny hats. "Well you try strolling 1&1/2 miles and see if you are tired" he pleaded with his overly concerned wife and mother.

Sleeping is another matter - it's getting better but slowly. I have moved to the bed (an upgrade from last week) but can't seem to get past the 1&1/2 hours at a time mark. It will come.

The kids are doing great - we all watched Amadeus this weekend (in an interesting way). Now how many people other than me did not know they print DVDs on both sides? Well, it seemed sort of an odd beginning and a short movie when we realized we watched the second half first.

Mom is still here. We decided that she would enjoy the doctor visit with us tomorrow. "Enjoy" may be a stretch but when the doctor takes out the 49 staples, she can think back on 49 things I did as a child (especially the things I got away with). Having her here has been great.

Today, I think I'll buy one of those Chia pets, rest a bit, try another bread recipe, update the beneficiaries on our life insurance policies, redo our investment portfolio, become a member of the Catholic Church, and begin training for the Boston marathon (that's Boston, Kentucky).

Next update - tomorrow after the doctor tells us the plan - actually I think we get to pick a plan but they can be pushy. Also on the agenda is to begin to work the second opinion from Stanford. We have a plan.

Thanks for all the support and well wishes. They mean a lot to me and Laura.

Love, Mike

Chapter 18

We've Been Through This Before

"Have a nice day."
- US Postal Service

In the fall of 1996 my father was diagnosed with pancreatic cancer. This may seem a bit out of place but nothing is out of place in my self-referential book. Pancreatic cancer is one of the most fatal forms of cancer with greater than 98% of patients dying within the first year. It is very common for the patient to die within a few months of diagnosis. I know they don't let you pick your cancer but if you ever get to choose, pick something else.

Dad's was a textbook case – start to finish. Dad never stood a chance. I'll never forget the refined bedside manner of the doctor when he told Dad, "Well Bob, we know what you're going to die from, unless you are lucky enough to be hit by a bus." We were shocked at the bluntness of the communication. Dad's response: "That's what I like about that Doctor."

Dad's last six weeks were not pleasant but he did get a good chance to say his goodbyes and make sure Mom was taken care of. He accepted his diagnosis and fate with honor and dignity. His focus was squarely on Mom, being sure that she was ready for the transition and a long life ahead - without him. He died peacefully one morning while I stood, soaking wet, in the shower in their bathroom. My brother, Ed, and I were both there (not in the shower).

That day brought several factors together in two unusually memorable moments. The hours after his death were memorable for being unexpected, inconsequential and really unforgettable.

The first thing we had to do was call the Hospice coordinator. We had been working with her over the preceding few weeks and, importantly, she had a plan. The Hospice coordinator had done this many times before and had a plan to take care of most things but much to my dismay, she asked me to help her get things started. She would take care of contacting the funeral home but she asked me to call the supplier of the home hospital bed, which had just been delivered two days earlier. We needed them to pick up the bed quickly to get it out of the middle of the living room. Hopefully they wouldn't respond too quickly and take the bed before the funeral home came to get Dad.

I called the delivery guy to arrange a prompt pickup and he asked, "Didn't I just deliver that bed the day before yesterday?" I confirmed that he had but informed him that we needed him to come back and get the bed right away because my father had passed away this morning.

His unthinking response (from the cab of his moving truck) was just two memorable words that kind of hit the nail on the head: "Bummer dude."

Later that day, the mailman brought a package to the door. He had delivered get-well cards each day of the previous six weeks and knew my father was sick. He asked my Mom how Dad was doing. Mom told him that Dad had passed away that morning. He expressed his sincere condolences and they exchanged the required, polite, and caring conversation.

When he turned to leave, he left Mom with one last parting phrase, "Have a nice day."

It sure gives you confidence in the US Postal Service and Hospice.

Chapter 19

Eye Contact

"If a bullfrog had wings, he wouldn't bump his ass."
- Robert Carter, my Dad

April 30, 2003

It's time for another update from the neighborhood. Yesterday's doctor visit actually started the day before when the doctor called to warm me up to the news he was going to give me on Tuesday. That's always a bad sign when the boss calls you in and says, "Here's what you will hear from me tomorrow." There are several reasons this doctor does this with me.

1) Phone calls make it slightly easier to avoid eye contact (this guy is a geek of monumental proportions - but a damn good one).

2) It gives me the time to read up in the medical textbooks and ask more "intelligent" questions.

3) It preps the family to avoid any extra screaming and yelling in the doctor's office.

The doctor visit included - reporting out on pathology. I'm a T2N3M0 Tonsillar Fossa Carcinoma case. We talked about the 9&1/2 hour surgery process. The doc made some good decisions like: find the tumor behind the tonsil - tonsil was clear, avoid the carotid artery, preserve that heart beat control nerve. It turns out - this doctor drinks Ensure during the procedure to keep alert. I should have asked him what flavor he drinks because all they do is make me gag. He could have gotten the tonsillar fossa tumor out with more margin but he would have had to take the carotid artery (and thus the entire patient) with it. So - a two-millimeter margin will have to do (for now). He may get the two-meter margin later.

Dr. Jansen approved the second opinion through the Stanford Tumor board. I had been struggling with getting Kaiser to pay for this - that's over. Kaiser had two options - pay for the Stanford *look or pay my psychiatric bills. If nothing else these second opinions are mental insurance - which is well worth anyone's money. I look at it as an $800 insurance policy or half a bottle of 2000 Chateau Petrus. Now - I get the Petrus.*

Dr. Jansen took out the staples. Their staple removers work very well on a numb patient. I took some Tylenol with codeine and didn't even need it. What a waste of 5 teaspoons of the good stuff.

After the doctor visit I had my first post-tonsillectomy restaurant experience. I ate the soup without gagging, hacking, coughing or throwing up. (We did ask for the corner table nearest the restroom just in case.) We wanted them to set up a visual and soundproof barricade but they just aren't that classy of a place.

We went in to visit the benefits office yesterday and get started in the paperwork process. It was nice to get out and show off my beauty scar. The one unexpected twist, I stopped in at work (just for a minute) to let people know I was still alive and not just an email ghost. I was wearing my new SpongeBob Square Pants shirt. The one advantage to being ill - no one even noticed the fashion faux pas. Wait till they see what I wear next time.

My shoulder has been very sore. I can't massage it out so we're trying heat and drugs. I have to be careful with the heat since I have no feeling in the skin in those areas. Basically – I need my wife to nurse me.

Mom heads back home today - that will leave a mark. She has "enjoyed" her visit (wrong word?). Laura and I have both appreciated her being here. This is not easy for her either. Going in with me to see the doctor (even though he has successfully avoided eye contact with us) has been good for her. The next appointment is with the radiation oncologist at Mt. Diablo Hospital on Tuesday. We will try to get to Stanford next week.

All in all, it is not too bad for a stage IV cancer guy. (This is not like the stage IV of the Tour d' France – Both are long and grueling but I have no cheering French people watching me).

More next time, Mike

Chapter 20

WTC

"The next time someone asks you if you are a god, say yes!"
- Ghostbusters

About two weeks after 9/11 we were called by the US Government to fly our sensors over the World Trade Center site in New York. The hope was that our sensors could aid in the recovery efforts at Ground Zero by mapping the hazardous gasses and potentially identifying locations of decaying bodies. We quickly got our equipment together, arranged for the aircraft and logistics at Teterboro airport in New Jersey and headed for the East Coast. Flying on United just after commercial air travel had restarted was different. The discussion in the first class cabin on that nearly empty flight to Newark centered on the change in attitude of the passengers following the successful passenger uprising on Flight 93. Never again would we go down without a fight! We had a "bring 'em on" attitude that one would not normally expect from naïve, middle-aged, upper-middle-class, white, Anglo-Saxon Protestants from suburbia.

The flight attendants had learned we were being deployed to the WTC site to aid in the rescue mission. One of them had lost two friends on one of the aircraft that had struck the WTC. They were very emotional and very glad to hear we were headed to NY to help. We ended up with four bottles of United's "Best Wine" in my carry off luggage. We'd break into three of those fine "vintages" over the next week. The last bottle I would lay to rest in my wine cellar as a remembrance (optimistic that it might get less bad with age).

On final approach to Newark we could see the still smoldering WTC site out the window. There was now a void where the twin towers had once stood. Our symbols of progress and civilization were gone along with thousands of innocent people.

I had two opportunities to visit the World Trade Center site during the recovery efforts. By visit, I mean, walk through the still-smoldering rubble. The emotion was overwhelming. The smallest things struck me hard: a woman's dress shoe, a signed piece of paper or a business card. It was the personal items that belonged to someone that stood out. Most of the debris was either part of the structure or unrecognizable fragments. The occasional recognizable items really personalized the impact of the calamity. These were the personal belongings of innocent victims.

At one point the cranes and trucks all stopped (as did we) - simultaneously. I asked our NYPD hosts (two brothers of a close friend from the lab) what had happened. This work stoppage was the normal site-wide response to the discovery of human remains. This was the real world. This was the site of the most significant battle in modern times between the future and the past. Between progress and stagnation. Between ancient religious zealots and the modern, civilized world. More than three thousand innocent victims lay silent in the rubble – victims of modern civilization's progress. This was not the site of the start of the war but this was the site of the first real "victory" for the other side. This was not our kind of war. Innocent civilians were not the targets of war. Civilized people worked to protect innocents from war. This opponent was not civilized. This war would be different. This war would take different methods to win. We were not prepared to fight this war. But this is a war we must win. The alternative is absolutely unacceptable for civilization.

We worked hard to understand the dangers in the recovery effort by mapping the gasses being released by the fire. There was fear that the Freon tank in the basement of the North Tower was leaking. The Freon was the coolant for one of the world's largest air conditioners and Freon leaking up through the burning rubble could be converted to toxic compounds (like phosgene). Such chemicals could provide ample opportunity for near-term, and long-term health effects (and law suits). I felt like we actually helped and it didn't take a long explanation to understand. I wanted to do more.

After our first visit to Ground Zero, we were taken to NYPD headquarters to brief the Police Commissioner on the plan for the support to the recovery effort. We had a team of about ten people all sitting in the Commissioner's conference room waiting for the 3:30 pm briefing time. We had arranged for a reservation at Tavern on the Green in Central Park at 6:00 pm. We had plenty of time we were sure.

The briefing began late with an unclassified version of the technology and the plan. They were interested. They continued to ask question after question about things that mattered to them (not so much to us). We could not do many of the things they would have really wanted (like locating decaying bodies or mapping the asbestos contamination down wind from the site). Some things are harder than others. We were pushing 5:00 pm and John Scarafiotti (Scarf), sitting in the back of the room, kept quietly pointing to his watch. If we were going to make 6 pm at Tavern on the Green I needed to wrap up. To get the reservation in the first place, Scarf had given the Tavern on the Green his credit card number. They explained that if we were no shows, his card would be charged $30 a chair. Everyone is so nice and friendly in the Big Apple.

This briefing was finally just thinking about wrapping up and it was 5:40 pm. We wouldn't get to the cars until 10 till 6 at the earliest (depending on the extent of the departure dance). Scarf was in panic mode. We explained to the NYPD and, one of "the boys" called the Tavern and explained as only a New Yorker could, "You're holding a reservation for a party of ten at 6 pm under the name of Scarafiotti? The Police Commissioner is discussing the recovery efforts with them. It would be a shame if anything happened to that reservation." Some things are easy. Now it's 6 pm and it must be a two-hour drive from downtown to Central Park in this traffic. The Police Commissioner offers a police escort up island. We start out with a patrol car (lights spinning and siren blaring) with our two minivans following headed through rush hour traffic up the East Shore Freeway under the Brooklyn Bridge toward the Upper East Side. Even Rush Limbaugh would have pulled to the side to avoid the wrath of the NYPD on a mission from God (Jake and Elwood would have been proud).

We know how Moses felt as the waters parted and he led his people to their Tavern in the Promised Land. It was like a scene from the Bourne Identity except they don't typically use mini-vans. Even Matt Damon in his future staring role in "The Carter Story" gets a stunt driver. Me – I'm on my own – with six scared colleagues shouting advice from the back pews. The problem is that every New Yorker is trained to in the art of "wake driving." They immediately cut in behind the police car and make their way through traffic in the wake. That "wake" is supposed to be us. We finally pick up a trailing NYPD vehicle – his siren blaring too. They can "wake" behind him.

What a ride! We finally get to Central Park and turn north up Central Park West. Flying up the parkway we sail right past Tavern on the Green. The lead cop, lights still flashing and siren blaring, realized his mistake about a block past the restaurant. He blocks traffic (all six lanes) and the entire caravan pulled a giant U-ie. We finally pulled in about 6:30 with his lights still spinning. We were rattled but – intact. I walk in with police escort and confirm the reservation was not lost and – we were greeted like we were truly important. They must have seen the caravan. I know I was impressed and shaken by the most dangerous and exhilarating drive in the history of failed-musicians-turned-physicists. (See page 314,159 of the "Guinness Book of World Records, Nerd Edition").

In character, but still in shock from the drive of my life, I head for the restroom. The hallway to the restrooms was very confusing (at least that's my story). They had mirrors up on the walls and – those damn Christmas lights created a cluttered illumination pattern. It's only October – do they have Christmas lights up all year long? Anyhow, confused and befuddled, I walk right into the Women's restroom. Sweet – couch and all. They really are nicer than the Men's restrooms.

Chapter 21

Popsicles

"I'm gonna make it!"
 - Many, including me

May 1, 2003

OK – two weeks have passed since the second surgery. In that time I have:

- Discovered the joy of modern medicine (any drug that ends in "ine" is good)

- Beaten back the phlegm gods (they still win a few battles but I'm winning the war). By the way – this is an epic battle between good and evil. Either you are with me or with the phlegm gods. If you aide, harbor, or finance them – I'll come after you too.

- Made eye contact with my surgeon one time. The best conversation we had was while he was looking in a microscope taking out my staples. And you guys thought I was a geek...

- Designated each of you a beneficiary (in the event that Laura and I and the kids and our parents, siblings, nieces, nephews, cousins and great aunt all die at the same time – you get the cash)

- Chosen the music for my daughter's wedding. Next week, I'm choosing the guy.

- Eaten 103 popsicles (yes – I'm counting – keeps my math skills fresh).

- Received 5 cookie bouquets, 8 books, 12 pints of ice cream, 42 balloons, 96 get well cards, 5 flower arrangements and a partridge in a pear tree. Feels like Christmas around here.

- Used 23 stamps on thank you cards alone (hey – I'm down to 77 stamps on my roll – still time to get in on the fun)

- Learned about nerves in the human body. What we know is – they have a mind of their own when bothered (just like my wife). This apparently will last me a while (just like my wife). I keep asking the doctor for a muscle relaxant – he keeps reminding me – the muscle has been removed. I blame that on him.

- Experienced the joy of an itchy beard. -- (Just found a new thing to complain about – this is fun). My previously mentioned daughter, to whom I religiously pay a weekly allowance for her services and affection says my beard looks "like a French woman's underarm." Needless to say, I am now holding half of her allowance until she at least changes the nationality. French?

- Taken 232 phone calls (and loved every one of them except the daily call from GMAC mortgage trying to get us to do something – I never let them finish the pitch – I tell them I'm recovering from surgery and I'm expected to die in a few weeks – that shuts them up in a hurry.)

The Doctor called on Friday (he has discovered the phone is a good way to interact without the threat of eye contact or a firm handshake). I made it through the tumor board. It was not clear whether Kaiser would recommend combined chemotherapy and radiation or just radiation therapy. Apparently, the chemotherapy drug of the day for this cancer is carboplatin. Carboplatin is apparently just as ineffective as cisplatin but has lower side effects. There are no data sets showing better results with combined chemo/radiation treatments but the doctors feel better doing both (Patients feel worse). The other big discussion is when do we put in the feeding tube, now or later? I vote now – If I get it in soon, I can save money by drinking cheaper wine.

My Mother-in-law and Father-in-law are coming out on Monday. Jean is a great cook so I've asked her to come out to fatten me up. I should hold off on the feeding tube until she is gone – her food is worth tasting.

The Department of Homeland Security, surgery, surgery, Mother-in-law, chemo, and radiation – what's next? – I'm thinking about *one of those role-playing adventure vacations to a Vietnamese prison camp.*

This next week we have appointments with a radiation oncologist (Tuesday), Stanford tumor board (Thursday) and the Kaiser Oncologist (Friday). I'll be looking for some sort of eye contact with one of these doctors. If I don't get some I'll think it's me. Maybe they just don't want to bond until they know I'm going to make it. Well, I'll tell them:

I'M GOING TO MAKE IT!

Love to all, Mike

[It turns out many of the "facts" in these letters are not really true. The chemotherapy drug of choice for squamous cell throat cancers is Cisplatin (Cisplatin has much more severe side effects than Carboplatin and therefore it must work better).]

Chapter 22

Grandma's House

"She Loves You Yeah, Yeah, Yeah."
- The Beatles

My Grandmother was different than most. Absolutely everything about her was special. To me and my brother, Grandma's house was the one place in the world where we seemed to be in charge. At Grandma's house we seemed to be the most important people in the world and in hindsight, we probably were.

Some of the memorable things my brother Ed and I liked to do were:

- Digging into the freezer in the basement for a cold Popsicle. She had one of those chest freezers that opened from the top. The popsicles were on the left – I could still find them today with my eyes closed.

- Throwing the ball up against the chimney and catching it over and over again. (They had a unique chimney where about half way up the brick stepped slowly in toward the roof like a small staircase.) This caused unpredictable bounces – just what two boys needed to keep them occupied for hours.

- Listening to the sound of her mantle clock in the living room when we slept over. To this day, when I hear a ticking clock in a quiet room, I think of her.

- Playing Parcheesi with my Aunt Sara. I would roll double sixes and count, "Onnneee, twoooo, threeee, no, let me start again. Onnneee, twoooo, threeee, wait, wait…" (Aunt Sara demands a note here in her defense – she is only 6 years older than me and as such should be thought of as a childhood near-peer not as an older, more mature member of the family – point made!)

- Seeing Aunt Sara get spanked when she lost in Parcheesi (this supposedly only happened once – I guess I just smiled and relived it in my mind over and over again.)

- Smelling fresh-baked homemade bread from Grandma's oven.

- Tasting her potato chip cookies.

- Playing in the basement – Grandma had a cool basement complete with Uncle Jack's bedroom.

- Helping Grandpa burn leaves in the back yard.

- Playing in the ditch between Grandma's house and the highway.

- Playing croquet in the back yard (sending Aunt Sara's ball way off into the weeds).

- Sled riding down the hill across the street.

- Eating what _we_ wanted for dinner – Grandma always seemed to know and always cooked the family meal with our tastes in mind. Memorable foods: roast beef and mashed potatoes, corn off the cob (frozen in the summer and re-warmed in the winter), barbequed chicken on the grill, potato chip cookies, goetta, and fish on Fridays.

- Taking family photographs with a camera on a timer.

- Watching slide shows with the portable screen in the living room (begging to see the Dam pictures - probably just so we could say the word "Dam").

- Playing with the Ouija board. (This was always played in the basement, away from the adults, for some Catholic reason).

- Picking walnuts from Grandma's walnut tree. I only remember eating the walnuts a few times but can still taste them. We shelled a lot of walnuts.

- Sitting in the shade of Grandma's maple trees. There were five or six huge soft maples in the backyard that dropped the helicopter maple seeds each year. We planted a few seeds from these trees in our yard as kids and they grew to be spectacular trees.

- Fearing the Ohio River floods. We were always trying to remember how high up the basement stairs the deepest flood had come (1963 or 1964). A little paint mark would have reduced the arguments. We do have one picture but it's not clear 40 years later if that was the high-water mark or not. If the house had been built in 1937, the entire house would have been under water.

- Admiring the cars. While we were stuck with a 1960 Chevrolet Corvair, a station wagon of some kind (luckily no wood paneling), two Chevy Novas and a yellow Chevy Beauville van (all with AM only radio), Grandpa Guild always seemed to get better cars – like the Mustangs from the early 60s and their legendary Ford Galaxy.

- Riding our bikes in Greenmound cemetery (that was one cool, old cemetery).

- Collecting knick-knack glassware for the collection displayed proudly in the front window.

- Wondering about the "Bridge and Turnpike Building Set" (This was our nickname for the Beckjord coal-burning power plant just downstream on the Ohio river from New Richmond).

- Sitting with Grandpa in his wooden rocking chair. Life was just slower and simpler back then.

Grandma finally passed away and the days that followed were difficult for all of us. She was the last of my Grandparents to pass on and this one was really different. I was her first grandchild. I was also her favorite – if you don't believe me - ask her! I always knew I was really special to her and she to me. I know my Mom, Brother, and Aunt Sara, and the many grandkids that followed felt the same. She had that way of making each us feel like we were her favorite. Only one of us was right – me.

We were all in Cincinnati helping make the arrangements and had just spent the morning at the Catholic Church in New Richmond working with the priest to be sure all was in order and she was really dead. Turns out – both were true.

On the way home, we stopped at the Skyline Chili in Cherry Grove for a three-way. A three-way is a plate of spaghetti, topped with Cincinnati Chili and grated cheddar cheese. (Served with a dish of oyster crackers on the side). Skyline Chili is truly one of the finer things in life. The four of us sat in the booth and were still numb and depressed with the loss of Grandma. At Skyline, there is little need for the formalities of a sit-down restaurant like "a menu." We all know what we want days before we walk in – a three-way and a Diet Coke. Aunt Sara, Mom and I order our three-ways like a broken record. The waitress turns to Ed. Ed orders – "A three-way and a cup of coffee." We all simultaneously burst out laughing! We had no idea Ed had EVER even drank a cup of coffee… sometimes, it's the little unexpected things you really remember.

Grandma was really, really special - may she rest in peace.

Chapter 23

What's Behind Door #3?

"Things are never so bad that they can't get worse."
  - Dr. Jay Zucca

May 9, 2003

Well, it's been three weeks since the second surgery. Time sure flies when you are learning to swallow. I've invented a new diet. It's a combination high-carb, low-carb diet. In one sitting you begin with all the high-carb food you can find (pastas, bread (soft), rice, etc.) You finish this off with a thirst-quenching Ensure. I find the Ensure typically needs a chaser and almost anything will do. Then I turn to a low-carb course (chicken or very easy to chew meat). You then follow this with a high-carb dessert – (ice cream, Popsicles, sorbet, cake (moist) etc.) Typically wait 1-3 minutes between diet courses if you wish to strictly follow this regimen. That is enough time to cleanse the pallet and prepare for full enjoyment of the food. Repeat as many times a day as possible. In one week I have gained back four pounds. Two weeks to go.

Doctors, doctors, doctors – this has been an interesting week. It began with a trip to a radiation oncologist (Dr. Chinn) at Mt. Diablo Hospital in Concord – a quick 45 minutes from home. They have a contract with Kaiser to irradiate people in need of high-energy photons. Dr. Chinn had treated a friend of mine and I too found him to be a great guy. He had been at the Kaiser tumor board on Friday the 2nd of May and heard my case. He argued for radiation only post-operative treatment course. (This is the big decision coming up – do I need radiation treatments alone or radiation with chemo). His opinion did NOT carry the day at Kaiser. He is proposing an all expenses paid, seven-week pass to paradise. Pass includes daily admission Monday through Friday (apparently cancer doesn't grow on the weekends or federal holidays). Sounds like the e-ticket rides are covered – 2 Gray's per day plus all the side effects. We had a very nice chat – lovely cup of hot tea – and departed still not knowing exactly what we were up against.

Wednesday was a fun day – no doctors on the schedule but we had to collect all my files for our trip to Stanford on Thursday. Luckily, we found some help in the head and neck surgery department. Alma coordinated what normally is supposed to take three weeks and we got this done in one day. Sometimes – you find the help you need, when you need it! Kaiser also had decided they did not want to pay for the second opinion from Stanford – Oh well – it is about the cost of a bottle of Chateau Petrus in a good year. On the other hand, there is a wine being sold in California that has been getting a lot of press. Some Charles Shaw vineyard cabernet. It's been selling for $1.99 a bottle. Its nickname is "Two Buck Chuck." At $24 a case – I could get 41.6 cases. Here's the review from the internet:

"And how is the wine? Well, it's not what I would call "good." On the other hand, it's not terrible. Let's call it a C minus. At two bucks a bottle, a C minus is a pretty reasonable return on investment. The Cabernet is the best of the lot. The finish is brittle, and the nose is from box-wine central, but there's enough red fruit on the mid-palate to make it acceptable, provided it is served with some food to mask its thinness."

Just like some of the stuff we drank at DHS... Sounds like wine for the feeding tube.

We went to Stanford Medical Center on Thursday: It was an interesting day. We show up at 7:45 to fill out a form (about three minutes) and wait for the doctors to arrive at 9:00. Stanford is more famous for their Marching Band than their processes. We get assigned a resident to "handle us" throughout the day – take my history, understand the case, and explain it to a parade of doctors to come in terms they can quickly understand.

Our resident leaves the room for a minute and I commented to Laura how much I liked her – Laura says, "That's because she's cute." I hadn't noticed (a sure sign of significant illness). Anyhow, the parade of doctors (and a few I didn't see (radiologist, *pathologist)) looked me over including the highly coveted "scope the nose and throat" procedure. They sent us away to wait in the cafeteria for another 1&1/2 hours while they rendered an opinion. The basic opinion from the Chairman of the Department (Dr. Goode) (in words appropriate for this distribution):*

- There are some uncertainties – run a few more tests (MRI, MRA, nasal biopsy) (The MRA is a magnetic resonance angiography – destined to look for potential damage the surgery might have done to my carotid artery. –That sounds important.)

- You are young and tough – prepare for combined chemotherapy and radiation – kill this now even if it makes you Miserable to do so. (That is a capital M in Miserable.)

- Don't forget to pay us.

- No – you cannot date the Residents.

Friday: It's back to Kaiser for an introduction visit to the oncologist. The oncologist is young and just my type (except he's the wrong sex and not that cute). He was not very familiar with my case so we brought him up to speed. He, as well as the radiation oncologist, would normally lean toward radiation alone following the surgery but they are open to alternate opinions.

Opinions – everyone has one. Ultimately, this will be a very difficult decision that Laura and I will have to live with (hopefully). There is not much (if any) data showing that adding chemotherapy helps with this particular form of cancer. The side effects are clearly substantially worse but if we're going to do it – now's the time. We have two weeks to decide (maybe less). Sometimes you feel like you are on Let's Make a Deal and being asked to trade it all for what's behind door number three. (Hope I end up with the lifetime supply of Pork and Beans.)

Next up – we need to schedule the MRI (Kaiser has accepted this recommendation from Stanford). We also need to get the nasal biopsy scheduled (also a Stanford recommendation), get the modeling and simulation for the radiation treatments started and gain more weight. Some of these are easier than others.

I'd like to thank everyone who has replied to these emails, sent cards, gifts, cash, and prizes and, of course, come to see me. Your thoughts, prayers and friendships are incredibly important to me - especially now. Thanks again – write and I will try to write back!

Love, Mike

Chapter 24

Dale (I mean "Mr. Swisher")

"That's Mr. Swisher"
- Dale Swisher

My high school had an awesome music program. I realized this in about the 6th grade when my parents took me to the Anderson High School rendition of "Annie Get Your Gun." In the pit was a full orchestra conducted by a young, vibrant conductor, Mr. Dale Swisher. I walked out and told my parents that I wanted to play in that orchestra someday. (I think they said – "you better practice.") There were several great music teachers at Anderson but the one that motivated me was Dale, (I mean Mr. Swisher.)

I joined the orchestra my freshman year and met Lou Proske and Alan Ropp. Lou and Al were both violinists (two years ahead of me) and the next thing I knew, we were forming a string quartet with Peggy Smotzer as our cellist. We were very good (for a high school string quartet) and – I learned my first viola joke!

The Al stories that emerged from our string quartet were priceless.

Al's family consisted of two parents, three boys, a younger sister and Martha. Martha was always home, typically in the living room standing, or sitting by the window. Martha wore something different every day, but she wasn't very active. Martha was a mannequin that the Ropp family treated just like a family member. Al would tell the neighborhood kids that Martha was his dead grandmother or his aunt suffering from arthritis (scared the neighbor kids to death).

One day our string quartet was practicing in Al's living room (with Martha listening carefully). Al spilled his coke on the carpeting. Instead of cleaning it up, Al just rearranged to furniture.

Once practicing at our house, while my mother was out at the store, Al replaced my mother's large indoor tree with a potted dead stick. (That original tree finally died just a few years ago after a very healthy 35 years.)

Our quartet played almost every Sunday morning at a local church (Salem Acres). The average age of the Salem Acres congregation was about 75. Every week we would walk away, well fed and with $50 to divide among the four of us. Plus, it got me to "church."

The key to the orchestra clan was the orchestra director, Dale (I mean Mr. Swisher). Dale (I mean Mr. Swisher) had very few rules; one was that we call him "Mr. Swisher." (Hence our tendency to call him Dale when he wasn't around). Dale (I mean Mr. Swisher) collected and nurtured talent. The best examples of that were Lou Proske and Alan Ropp. Lou had perfect pitch (a rare and awesome trait) and could play the violin with the best of them. Lou was the concertmaster of the orchestra and had a very unique style. Al was the 1st chair second violinist and an incredibly diverse talent. Al was also a composer and during his senior year, composed a two-violin and flute concerto that was performed with full orchestra accompaniment at our high school graduation at Music Hall in Cincinnati. This was one talented guy. Al was also a guy that thought rules were made for him to break. He was the ringleader, the troublemaker and the inspiration. There was only one Al (and the world is better for that).

Al was always up to something. Every day at the same time, our school's vice principal, Bill Stephan, would leave his office and make the rounds walking around school. Every day, at that same time, Al would call the vice principal's office and his Asian secretary would answer. (This story is so politically incorrect in today's world but suburban Cincinnati at the time was very mono-cultural. Our idea of diversity was Methodists and Presbyterians sharing the lunch table). Every day the secretary would answer the phone and Al would ask for Bill. Her response was always the same: "I so sorry, Bill no here now." We would all listen and laugh. She never caught on.

We "ruled" the orchestra room (wow – sounds so stupid). Dale (I mean Mr. Swisher) had an office with two doors, one leading to the hallway, one leading onto the orchestra room. His office was almost never locked. When he did lock the doors, Al couldn't get in to call the Vice Principal's office at the defined time and we didn't feel like we were the "rulers." But a locked door never stopped Al.

One day, locked out of Dale's (I mean Mr. Swisher's) office, Al pulled a table up against the door, stacked another table on top of that and a chair on top of the second table. Al climbed up the pile, pushed up a ceiling tile and made his way over the door jam and dropped down into Dale's (I mean Mr. Swisher's) office. He unlocked the door, he made the phone call to Stephan's office and we ruled again. In the process of doing this, he broke the ceiling tile on the inside of Dale's (I mean Mr. Swisher's) office, just above the door. He carefully replaced the tile and one could barely see the crack. That tile was still broken 10 years later when I returned to visit Dale (I mean Mr. Swisher).

Times were good. We all knew our favorite composers, violinists and pieces. We had a great place to hide from the jocks. Many of the kids in our high school went on to be professional musicians or music teachers. We all shared one important thing, a real respect for Dale (I mean Mr. Swisher).

Chapter 25

The 4-week Mark

"Pain is inevitable but misery is optional."
- Barbara Johnson

May 16, 2003

It's time for a week-four update. This week has been quite eventful with such highlights as – I slept through the night for the first time, I got bolted to a table and interrogated and I was visited by wise men (and woman) from the east. Want to find out more? – Read on.

You will recall from the last update that my in-laws were in town. I decided to work them like slaves (remember I can't pick up anything heavier than two Kleenexes (spelling of the plural of Kleenex alludes me to this day)). They painted the living room, tore out and rebuilt an old section of fence, cleaned and cleaned, cooked, transported the kids, mowed the yard, planted flowers, cooked some more and then, finally, they went home. It was great to have them here – we needed the work done. Doctor says, "If you can survive a week and a half with your mother-in-law, the chemo will be easy." (He's never eaten her cooking – she's easy!)

The rest of the week was filled with doctor appointments. On Sunday morning I got a call from Kaiser asking me if I could come in that morning for my MRI (the one that Stanford recommended for me). We scheduled a time just before lunch and they immediately called back and asked to reschedule (apparently, their technician didn't feel comfortable with me – and they hadn't even met me yet) – so it was scheduled for dinnertime (the second shift personnel were sleeping and couldn't reject me).

For those of you who are claustrophobic – feel free to skip to the next paragraph. Those MRI's are not as easy as they sound – even for a former spelunker. They strip you of all metal, lay you down, stuff some ear plugs in your ears, clamp on a face guard and tell you to hold perfectly still – for an hour! Oh, and you in a tube the size of a wastepaper basket. For a guy having swallowing problems this was just enough to push me to the edge. After 40 minutes, they pulled me out, dropped 1/8 tsp of water in my mouth and 1/4 cup of Gadolinium in my vein and pushed me back in. A little Valium would have been better. I finally emerged, grumpy and ready to go home. (This test will prove to be important later in the week.)

The Monday morning trip was to the dentist. Uneventful – they took 20 x-rays – nothing compared to what's to come. My dentist pointed out that when he was in school, they would routinely pull all the teeth of someone in my situation. Thank God he's old and the treatments have advanced. I've started brushing my teeth 6 times a day as a precaution (and I'm scared). On Monday afternoon, we traveled to the radiation center in Concord only to have our radiation planning appointment canceled because the MRI had not been read yet. If nothing else, we're learning the route to Mt. Diablo medical center.

On Tuesday, I met with Drs. McCarthy, Stoutland, Wheeler and Wadsworth. We discussed multiple treatment options including cabernet-based therapies (for taste bud stimulation) and single-malt-based treatments (good for whole body relaxation). My alcohol consumption is down to sniffing and the occasional 1/8-teaspoon swig. I've turned to enjoying it by watching the facial expressions of others. This set of holistic scientists worked with me all evening and the following afternoon with the dramatic result – Wednesday night was my first whole night's sleep in over a month!

On Thursday, we were back off to the rescheduled radiation-planning meeting. I had not done quite enough reading to prepare me for this so, my anxiety was artificially low. Step 1 – change clothes into one of those "see my back side" gowns (I look good in those). Step 2 – lay on hard flat table with exceptionally uncomfortable neck rest. Step 3 – strap a hot, wet, deformable mask to my face and bolt me down to the table. Step 4 - strap my arms down (connected to my feet) to pull the shoulders down as far as possible. About this time I realize my radiation technician has been trained in the Vietnamese prison system. She tells me,

"You'll be bolted to the table for the next hour. I hope you like elevator music." I prefer Barry Manilow but – she didn't ask.

Over the next hour, I was: drawn on by a permanent marker, probed with lasers and x-rays, given three tattoos (one love dot for my wife and each kid). I also had serious eyelash issues. I was bolted down so tightly that I couldn't open my eyes but my eyelashes (being particularly long and beautiful) were penetrating out from underneath the plastic mesh mask – not a problem until they apply tape, make some kind of measurement and then rip the tape off. I may not have experienced childbirth (except as a baby) but I have now had an eyelash pluck. Men are such wimps.

As the end of the session nears, my radiation oncologist comes in the room. I'm about ready to learn that he took the "Bedside Manner 101" (BM-101) class pass/fail. You can guess his grade later. He tells me that the results of the MRI are in. Now remember, I'm bolted to the table – shoulders pulled toward the feet. My eyes and mouth are forced shut under the mask and that damn elevator "relaxation music" is echoing in my ears (where's Barry when you really need him?).

He tells me, "Hey – they found another tumor in your lkxdjial node. We've decided on your treatment. You are doing the chemo and radiation." I ask him (as best I can from under the mask) – "Can we talk about this in a minute?" His response – "Oh! – Sure." He just took the final exam – PASS!

The good news is, it was not the lkxdjial node like I first heard him say – It's some other hard to remember thing – the parapharyngeal node (just like Stanford suspected!). The really good news is – They found it! We were about to decide on the radiation-only therapy. This diagnosis makes the decision for us – it's the combined radiation/chemotherapy treatment (followed by more chemotherapy). Thank God we went to Stanford!

They also found a souvenir – The surgeon had left one of the staples in my neck. My son Dave had seen it a few days earlier but I had told him he was crazy.

After a meeting with my wise men from the east (another Dr. – Dr. McQueary), I had another great night sleep Thursday night. No sense losing sleep over a node you can't even pronounce.

Friday took me back to the surgeon (to remove the staple). And yes – a $10 co pay was required to get the last staple out. The surgeon got another chance to scope me (run that fiber optic in the nose and down the throat). I really enjoy that one. He reviewed the MRI – made some comments about the radiologists spending only 3 years in residency (versus his 7). He said, "Radiologists have issues." Now that's one hip surgeon. We're still debating the diagnosis.

Looks like more opinions are in order – I'm seeing another surgeon on Monday and off to UC Davis for a 6th opinion on Friday. In the meantime – treatments are scheduled to start on Tuesday, May 27th. They are closed on Monday the 26th – cancer doesn't grow on weekends or federal holidays.

I turn 45 on Friday the 30th. May 30th, 2008 will be both my 50th birthday and my 5-year cancer survival date. I know it's one day at a time but – that will be a hell of a birthday party. I hope you all join me – it'll be at our place – 4pm.

I'd again like to thank everyone who has replied to these emails, sent cards, gifts, cash, and prizes and, of course, come to see me. Your thoughts, prayers and friendships are incredibly important to me - especially now. Thanks again – write and I will try to write back!

Sorry this update is so long – too much funny stuff happened this week.

Love, Mike

Chapter 26

Drive-by Viola Recital

"I love playing the Viola. It's like taking a vacation."
  - Lou Proske (professional violinist)

Once upon a time in a far away land, Al Gore invented the World Wide Web for a reason – the world needed a viola joke web site. Viola players are one of the classic jokes of the world. "Violinists that couldn't make it" is the normal rap but there is so much more. They are one of the few "unprotected classes" in today's society. Fill out "viola player" on a job application and see how often you get the interview. There is so much unfair profiling going on in the classical music world. Justified? You be the judge. So here goes – from memory:

What is the difference between a violin and a viola? The viola burns thirty minutes longer.

How do you know if you have perfect pitch? If you can throw a viola into a dumpster from ten paces without hitting the rim.

What is the difference between a viola and a chain saw? About an octave.

Did you hear about the new crime wave in New York City? Drive-by viola recitals.

Why do you never leave a viola in the back seat of an unlocked car? Someone may break in and leave another viola.

Do you know the four members of a standard string quartet? A good violinist, a bad violinist, a former violinist, and someone who hates violinists.

What do good violists keep in their viola case? A violin.

What do good violists keep in their viola case? No one knows, they haven't found a good violist.

What's the definition of an optimist? A violist with a pager.

What's the definition of a masochist? A violist with perfect pitch.

What's the definition of a sadist? A violist with a bow.

What do you do with a dead violist? Move him back a stand.

A corollary joke in physics: What do you do with a dead high-energy physicist? Move him down on the author list. (I hope you are a physicist and get that one – it's really a good one… trust me.)

How did the composer get the violist to play up-bow staccato? He wrote a whole note and labeled it "solo." (My favorite)

What do you call someone that hangs around with musicians? A Violist.

How much does the perfect violist weigh? About six ounces, not including the urn.

How much does the perfect violist weigh? Sqrt(-1)*150 pounds - (The perfect violist is imaginary.)

How do you get two violists to play the same note? Shoot both of them.

What does a school for the deaf and a great viola have in common? They both have mutes.

What's the difference between a Viola and a '57 Chevy? You can tune a '57 Chevy.

What do Violists use for birth control? The recital.

A freshman comes home after his first year in college and tells his parents, "I've got something important and difficult to tell you. After a difficult freshman year away at school, I have finally found myself. After many struggles and much self reflection, I finally realize, I'm a gay violist." His parents respond in shock "Violist?"

What's the difference between a harpist and a violist? A harpist spends 90 percent of the time tuning and 10 percent of the time playing out of tune. A violist plays out of tune 100 percent of the time.

When you hear a violist playing Beethoven's Für Elise, you know they are just practicing their trills.

Next year's hit video game (modeled after Guitar Hero) – Viola Hero… To get a perfect score you can't move the bow.

Or… My son David's version of Viola Hero… It's an urban sniper game where you roam the city picking off the Violists without injuring the other musicians.

Chapter 27

Kathy Lee Gifford Sings Love Songs

"Get The Comfy Chair!"
- The Spanish Inquisition, Monty Python's Flying Circus

May 24, 2003

This was a relatively quiet week on the medical front. No real news from the doctors (and thus nothing very funny either). I did visit Dr. Fong (a head and neck surgeon at Kaiser) for a second opinion on the MRI scan. He agreed that the tumor in unpronounceable region (parapharyngeal node) was there, big and inoperable. He did note that surgery was possible if chemotherapy and radiation failed but the description of the procedure sounded a lot like getting strapped to the tracks and run over by the train. Believe it or not, there appears to be something worse than chemotherapy and radiation to the mouth and throat.

On Wednesday, we visited the oncologist who apologized for not getting a hold of us before the news was broken to us last week about the new tumor. He actually talked to us without strapping me down. He reviewed the near term plan (three chemotherapies, day 1, 22 and 43; and seven weeks of radiation) and the follow-up plan (four months of chemo following the chemo-radiation). He "thinks" we can get through this follow-up chemo but is not sure. I only see three ways to "not get through" the treatment and all of them seem pretty bad:

1) I quit (not good)

2) They quit because they think I'm not going to make it (not good) and

3) They quit because I don't make it (really not good).

The only "good" option I see is to get through it! He reiterated the "no-pain, no-gain" theory of combined chemotherapy-radiation treatments. I call it the "the more miserable you are, the better" plan. I suggested we add leeches and a few good bloodlettings (they have been used in the past and they really hurt). He was less than amused. He continues to inform me that this is going to be rough. I continue to tell him "I'm tough." He thinks he's right. So am I.

On Thursday, we got our first "test zap" at the radiation center. I found myself bolted back to the table under the facemask. This time – it was a short twenty minutes or so. I forgot to bring my "Kathy Lee Gifford Sings Love Songs" CD. I figure if I'm miserable, they should be too! I actually own that CD (thanks to my wife's prank valentine's gift a few years ago). Frank and I have the only two known copies in existence.

On the personal front, this has been a fantastic week. I'm gaining weight (I think I gained a whole one pound). It's not as easy as it used to be to gain weight – a complaint I'm sure I share with no one. My Aunt Sara spent the week with us driving the kids around, answering the phone, reading my mail and eating lots of great food! My Brother arrived back in California for a weekend visit on Thursday night. We've finished the fence repair and are now working on a table in the wood shop. We all took the ferry to San Francisco on Saturday and had a really nice afternoon looking at wacky hats for me to wear when my hair falls out.

The highlight of my week was the birthday party lunch on Thursday. It was attended by almost two hundred of my closest friends and was one heck of a good time! I can't tell all of you how much your friendship and support means to me. There are no words to describe the feelings. The things people will do to humiliate me in public continue to astound me. Just remember – when I get better, I'll get even.

Another highlight hit us on Friday when we returned from our weekly dinner at the Clowers' – (yeah – they get to humiliate me weekly). In the mail was a hand written, get well note from Tom Ridge. Tom and I have met twice now and let me tell you – he's a politician and he's good! I call him "Tom." He calls me "Hey security! What's he doing here?" We're close.

Chemotherapy (cisplatin) starts on Monday with a six-hour session in the comfy chair. I already have every anti-nausea prescription known to man. Taking all those will make you sick to your stomach. Radiation treatments start on Tuesday. I should get the feeding tube this week or early next (no schedule yet for that). This is the start of the second climb. The first few weeks are supposed to be relatively easy. I'll let you know next weekend how "easy." Until then – keep up the positive vibes. I feel them and I need them.

Love, Mike

Chapter 28

Lazt Chair, Columbuz Zymphony

"Zink about it!"
- Professor Georges Janzer, Indiana University School of Music

For those of you who haven't picked this up, I'm a physicist. Let me start by saying, I have not always been a physicist. Once upon a time in a far away land I was an excellent viola player (the musical equivalent to Army Intelligence). I auditioned and was accepted to attend college as a music major at Indiana University in Bloomington, Indiana. I was accepted as a performance major (i.e. I thought I was really good). I turned down a full scholarship at S.E. Missouri State (music major) to attend IU. IU was (and still is) considered the best music school in the nation (some under-informed, east-coast snobs consider it number two to Julliard). The debate continues just like the Ohio State-Michigan, Duke-North Carolina, Cal-Stanford, and Cal Tech-MIT rivalries. By all assessments, it is a great music school. Plus IU consistently kicks Julliard's butt in basketball (even after the departure of Bobby Knight). You should see those little Julliard music nerds try to dunk.

I had auditioned and been assigned to the top Viola instructor (Georges Janzer) and joined the top orchestra at IU (there were five full concert orchestras – it's a really big music school). Georges Janzer was from the old country, Austria, and had a very thick, Edward-Teller-like accent. Georges was as famous as you get for a real Violist. Pinky Zuckerman is more "famous" and has more recordings but he's a violinist impersonating a violist – it's a subtle detail but important to the studied violist (please see the section on viola jokes).

I worked hard that freshman year. I practiced every day (typically at night) and became an excellent pinball player. There was only one pinball machine worth playing – Fireball. For the pinball major, there was nothing better. You could get three pinballs going at once and the flippers could be finessed and controlled like no other machine. It was not unusual to drop in a quarter and play all night, leaving many free games to subsequent players after I got tired of playing. I also minored in Space Invaders - the first really good video game.

I also played a lot of viola. Getting a practice room was always a challenge so every evening, after dinner, I made my way to the pinball parlor, played for a few hours, and then headed to the music building to play until the wee hours of the morning. Other classes I took included: sight singing, ear training, piano, orchestra, and math for idiots (M118). The big class (six credit hours) was my viola lesson with Georges Janzer. Georges was absolutely awesome – breaking the mold that viola players were just rejected violinists. He could make the viola sing. Of course, he played one of the finest string instruments in the world – an Italian Amati viola from the late 1500s.

Near the end of the year at one of my lessons, Georges was frustrated with me as he attempted to improve my technique. At the end of the lesson Georges said, in his thick Austrian accent, "Mike, ve muzt talk." Georges was holding his priceless Amati viola and his $10,000 Tourte bow (a lot of money for a bow at the time).

Georges goes on to say, "Mike, Zere are two reazonz ve accept people into zee school of muzic. Von is becauze zey are GREAT! Two is becauze, ve need za money. Zink about it." I was stunned – like a viola player playing a solo in concert.

He went on to say, "I Zink you vork two, three more yearz, you make lazt chair Columbuz Zymphony... Columbuz, Indiana."

I got ze message. In a daze, I walked down to the University registrar's office to change my major. I stepped up to the counter and began to answer questions to fill out the form to change my major to something that would ultimately free me from the cozy, melodious futures of Columbuz, Indiana. The conversation started out very pleasant:

"What's your name?"

"Mike Carter" (note the lack of stuttering… I'm developing some self confidence.)

"What's your major?"

"Music."

"What do you want to change your major to?"

"Undergraduate Division, Undecided!" I declared. (This is the major for all freshmen at IU unless they auditioned and were accepted into zee school of muzic).

Her answer caught me by surprise, "Oh, we have a rule at Indiana. Once you have a major, you can't change back to undecided. You have to pick another major."

Well, Shit! I didn't know that. I stood there and said, "OK, well, jeez, I guess, Um, Um, Um, I really liked my physics teacher in high school. Put down physics."

She said, "I don't think you can just 'put down physics.'"

"Why not?" I asked.

She leaned forward across the counter and whispered, "Because it's really hard."

"Do you have a list of what I can 'put down'?"

"Not really." she said. "Actually, my best friend is a secretary in the Physics Department, why don't you go over and talk to her about being a physics major."

Determined to take yes for an answer, I walked over to Swain Hall, found her best friend, told her my story, and asked her, "Can I be a physics major?"

She replied quite thoughtfully, "A few years ago we had a student who was a double major in physics and music. I hear they go together. I think you can do it."

Back I went, telling the clerk at the registrar's office, "Your friend said I can do it."

"OK," she said. And the next thing I knew, I was a physics major.

The next big challenge – how do I tell my Mother? My Mom, bless her heart, is cost-conscious, monetarily constricted, fiscally conservative, cash-flow-challenged, spending-averse, savings-empowered; read "tight." It turns out that not many of my music credits were going to transfer over to a degree in physics. I tried to talk them into using sight reading and sight singing as a foreign language but – guess what – they were not amused. Ear Training, Sight Singing, Piano, Viola, Music Theory, Orchestra – all pretty useless as a physics major. Even my Math credit (M118 – math for idiots - in which I had gotten a B) was essentially useless. I thought my explanation of the B was both reasonable and accurate – "I didn't even bother to go to the stupid class it was so easy." Again – they were not amused. A sense of humor was not big in the physics department prior to my arrival.

Mom and Dad had paid out of state tuition plus room and board for a year so that I could learn how to play Fireball! And let me tell you, I was good… I called my Dad. He was immediately 100% supportive (not knowing the Fireball thread). I don't think he was surprised. He said, "you're doing the right thing. Don't worry about your Mother. I'll take care of her." With the undying support of my father, it was done.

I had "failed" at something for the first time. "Failed" is not an event, "failed" is an emotional state. My Mom and Dad were there to save me. To protect me from "total failure." It is really important to not just "be able to fail" but to actually experience "failure" and recover. Once you recover, "failure" is empowering! Knowing that "failure" is not fatal is emotionally enabling. Everyone should do it. You often here people say "fail early and fail often" but do they really mean, fail emotionally? Knowing in your heart that it really is OK to fail and recover frees you from the burden of never being able to fail. It should be everyone's goal to fail and recover at least once – and I suggest early life failures are preferred. It will change your life for the better.

Failing was the best thing that could have happened to me – Thankz to George Janzer for making the call and thanks to Mom and Dad for enabling my recovery. What else should great professors and great parents do?

Chapter 29

Let's Get this Party Started

*"Be careful about reading health books,
you may die of a misprint."*
- Mark Twain

May 31, 2003

Well, we're started. One chemo and four radiation treatments down! For some reason, I always use the plural (we) knowing that I'm not the only one suffering. If you've ever had to deal with me as a "sick" person, you know I take great effort to make sure everyone around me suffers as well. This week started with a wonderful day of chemotherapy and ended with a birthday/anniversary party I won't forget. From the beginning: The chemo treatment was uneventful. They started me with an IV and put me on the drip for about three hours. They call it a "drip." It was more like a flow. They try to get a lot of liquids in you because the cisplatin is tough on the kidneys. Well, there was a pregnant woman between me and the restroom – boy was she sorry. I have no idea how many times I elbowed her to get to the kidney relief station. My brother, Ed, and I sat and told stories from the "good old days." The nurses were great except that they had already heard all my jokes. I came home with enough anti-nausea drugs to make you sick to your stomach.

Tuesday wasn't too bad. I reached a local maximum in my weight – 177 (all due to the pregnant woman obstructing my route to the restroom). This weight situation would soon change. We had our first irradiation on Tuesday. I did notice that the only "we" in the room was ME! Where's all that "help" when you need it? I am developing an aversion to the taste of 6 MeV Gamma rays. They taste like you are biting on lead-lined duct tape (just like we used to do in the Nuclear Test Program).

The radiation treatments consist of getting bolted to the table, neck in the most uncomfortable position, head down under the mask, laser shined in the eye (I hope this is a class one laser – safety first), arms strapped to your feet. The technicians scream, "run for your lives" as they evacuate the room and hit the ON button. It's about 22 seconds on each side of the neck and 40 seconds to the upper chest. We can do this.

Wednesday was a little different. Judy Kammeraad had warned me that the third day of chemo was the worst. I hope she was right. Wednesday was the ultimate, low energy, no appetite day. We did have a doctor's appointment with the GI surgeon. It's always nice to meet a new doctor. This guy, Dr. Fredman, was a character right out of a Woody Allen movie. We're trying to work my feeding tube insertion around my white blood cell count and his vacation (probably to Palm Springs). We're scheduled for the 12th of June. The way I felt today, I don't need a feeding tube – I'm FULL! That $500 anti-nausea drug almost worked. (I also lost three pounds today – go figure). After the GI appointment we went and got the second radiation treatment. Again, I was alone in the room. I'm sensing a pattern developing.

As of Thursday I had lost more weight. Maybe it was just water? My appetite is slowly returning. The key word is slowly. I'm continuing to work on building a serving table for the dining room. Work in the woodshop is very slow (slower than I am normally). I feel like I'm running at 50 Hz instead of 60.

We finally received the written opinion from our Stanford visit on May 8th. It was only 21 days to get an opinion on a treatment that I've already started (their people talked to our people). The Stanford results contained some interesting information. I quote: "Generally, this is a well-appearing gentleman in no distress." (I tell you – I think the resident took a liking to me – I should have dressed better and not taken my wife). They mention a "large crater at the right tonsillar fossa." I should have majored in astronomy. Also noted: "the patient denies any tobacco use and drinks approximately two glasses of alcohol per week." The key word here is "approximately." There is a bunch of other medical stuff that makes me sound like I have issues.

Friday was the last day of the week again this week. We received a video birthday card from my friends in DC (at the Department of

Homeland Security). They had no trouble getting the camera through the security checkpoint at the office. The guards just stared into the camera – stunned – and let the film crew walk right in. Thanks Sonya Bowyer! It was awesome! I can't wait to move into my cubicle at 7th and Dump. The fourth radiation treatment went as expected – by myself again.

Upon returning home, we found the kids and all their friends decorating our house for my birthday (and mine and Laura's anniversary (#22)). We had a houseful (15) and a great time. I struggled through reading the birthday cards (they say the chemo makes men act pregnant (emotionally)). I break into tears just opening the envelopes. So I find out Britney and Justin have broken up and I'm in the bathroom for thirty minutes. Poor Justin.

With the support of my friends and family, I'm going to make it! We're taking volunteers to join me in the gamma ray room or to shave their heads in sympathy. Photoshop "enhanced" entries are welcome but will only get half credit.

Until next week, keep the emails coming. I may not respond to every one of them but I'll probably cry when I double click on them - hey - it's like I'm pregnant without the weight gain!

Love, Mike

Chapter 30

Speaking of Nerds

"A joke is a very serious thing."
- Sir Winston Churchill

I have developed a strange affinity for "nerd jokes." This has become a useful tool in differentiating myself and my like-kind from the pretenders – the non-nerds. If you get more than a couple of these jokes, you might be a nerd too. Read ahead at your own peril.

This obsession for the perfect nerd joke started on the first day of college physics at Indiana University in 1977 (a year that will not live in infamy). If anyone can name something significant that happened in 1977, please feel free to waste your breath. (Oh – I have one - I met my wife – Nope – 1978 – See! Nothing! (Unless you count the discovery of the rings of Uranus on March 10th, or the premier of Star Wars on May 25th, or the first Apple II sales on June 5th, or the launch of Voyager II on August 12th, or the first flight of the then-secret F-117A (stealth aircraft) on December 1st). It was a slow year for most but a good year for nerds.

What is the "perfect" nerd joke? The perfect nerd joke depends on the audience. Like all nerds, the teller must study his victims, understanding not only their graduate educations and specialty fields but also the fields of their collaborators as wisdom and humor are sometimes transmitted by osmosis. Knowing the field, one must choose the jokes wisely. A good nerd joke is one that when told in a large audience receives a subtle hush from the audience except for the laughter of a handful of nerds in the audience. A "great" nerd joke even discriminates between the nerds with the nerdiest getting the joke and the "pretenders" left behind. The "perfect nerd joke" is received with hushed silence but for the outburst of laughter from the one and only one nerd in the audience. Not till then, is perfection found. It's sure sweet when you hear it.

To give an example of a "good nerd joke" executed poorly, I recall the story of a talk I gave at an International Neutrino Physics Conference. I was talking about the utility of anti-neutrinos in National Security Programs. Anti-neutrinos are sub-atomic particle of antimatter with an unknown but very, very small rest mass. When the neutrino was "invented," Enrico Fermi was quoted as saying "I have made the mistake of postulating a particle that can never be detected." We, the scientific community, did finally learn how to detect them even though they barely interact with matter. Neutrinos are a very niche field in physics – antineutrinos even more so.

We had figured out a way to use antineutrinos to monitor nuclear reactors. But back to my talk: It was sweet. I always try to start my talks with one good physics/nerd joke but I knew that this would be a rough audience. I told one of the jokes below (I don't remember which one) and the entire audience laughed. I then solicited the members of the audience to come up with a good neutrino joke. They were quiet until one member of the audience got up and said, "A nubar ran in to a guy." The audience erupted in laughter (this is apparently THE classic neutrino physicist joke... there are about fifty people in the world that get this one, and every one of them was in the room.)

To discover how big a nerd you are read ahead: (if you need explanations, you are likely not a nerd and you can sleep well.)

What do you get when you cross a blueberry with an elephant? Blueberry elephant sine theta.

What do you get when you cross a blueberry with a mountain climber? Zero, a mountain climber is a scalar.

A physicist, mathematician and an engineer are all asked the same question: "Are all odd numbers prime?" The mathematician answers, "Well, 1's prime, 3's prime, 5's prime, 7's prime... therefore, by induction, all odd numbers are prime." The physicist answers, "Well, 1's prime, 3's prime, 5's prime, 7's prime, 9's not prime, 11's prime, 13's prime... so – within experimental error, all odd numbers are prime." The engineer answers, "Well, 1's prime,

3's prime, 5's prime, 7's prime, 9's prime, 11's prime, 13's prime…"

Heisenberg is pulled over for speeding. The officer comes up and taps on the window. Heisenberg rolls down the window and the officer asks him, "Sir, do you have any idea how fast you were going?" Heisenberg answers, "No, but I know exactly where I am!"

What do engineers use for contraception? Their personalities.

So Einstein gets on Amtrak the other day and asks the conductor, "Does Chicago stop at this train?"

The waters finally receded and Noah walked the animals off the arc and instructed each of them to "Go forth and multiply. I'll be back next year to see how you are doing at restoring your flocks." A year later Noah returned and observed flocks of geese, families of ducks, herds of antelope, crowds of people and finally came across a pair of snakes. Noah asks the snakes, "Where are all your young ones?" The pair of snakes replied, "We didn't know how to 'go forth and multiply,' we're adders." Noah said, "I have an idea, you need a more comfortable home, then you will feel more comfortable multiplying." Noah goes into the forest with his axe and returns with arms full of logs and builds them a log cabin, with log furniture, and log accessories. When he finished, he left them again with a promise to return the next year to ensure their species was thriving. The next year, Noah returned to see a thriving community of snakes with young snakes everywhere, He asked the snake-parents, "How did you do it?" They replied, "As adders, it was easy to multiply once we had our log tables."

DeBroglie and Maxwell went to a baseball game. Once an inning de Broglie quickly stood up raised his hands and sat back down. Finally a fan behind them yelled, "What are you doing buddy? – SIT DOWN!" Maxwell replied, "Leave him alone, he's doing the particle."

A physicist, a biologist and a mathematician are sitting in a café talking and sipping coffee. An FBI agent walks in and asks for their help. "I need to know how many people are in the building across the street. I'll return later. Please keep an eye on the building." Time passes and they see two people walk into the building. A little later they see three people come out. The FBI agent returns and asks them "OK, how many people are in the building?" The physicist replies, "Two people went into the building and three emerged, we need more data, we cannot yet determine..." The biologist interrupts, "It's obvious, two people went into the building, they reproduced, then emerged from the building..." The mathematician interrupts, "Wait a minute. We just need one more person to go into the building, then it will be empty."

An engineer, a physicist and a statistician go hunting. After walking much of the day, they finally see a deer in the distance. The engineer says, "Give me the gun, I'll calculate the trajectory." He takes careful aim calculating the range, speed of the bullet and the force of gravity. He fires "Bang!" "Missed – two feet to the right." The physicist grabs the gun and says, "You forgot to correct for the wind speed." He takes careful aim, this time correcting for the wind. "Bang!" "Missed – two feet to the left." The statistician shouts, "Got him!"

How do you tell if a statistician is lying? His pencil is moving.

Why did God invent economists? To make meteorologists look good.

How did the physicist learn to sleep on the bed of nails? He started sleeping on one nail and worked his way up to the whole bed.

Did you hear about the scientist that got a divorce? His wife caught him carbon dating an older woman.

What do you do with a dead high-energy physicist? Move him down on the author list.

How do you get 300 high-energy physicists on the back seat of a Volkswagen? Tell them it's a Phys Rev Letter author list.

An experimentalist comes running excitedly into a theorist's office, waving a graph taken off his latest experiment. "Hmmm," says the theorist, "That's exactly where I'd expect to see that peak. Finally, after all these years, data that validates my theory." In the middle of it, the experimentalist says, "Wait a minute," studies the chart for a second, and says, "Oops, this is upside down." He turns it over. "Hmmm," says the theorist, "That's even easier to explain."

What is the difference between a physicist, an engineer, and a mathematician? If an engineer walks into a room and sees a fire in the middle and a bucket of water in the corner, he takes the bucket of water and pours it on the fire and puts it out. If a physicist walks into a room and sees a fire in the middle and a bucket of water in the corner, he takes the bucket of water and pours it eloquently around the fire and lets the fire put itself out. If a mathematician walks into a room and sees a fire in the middle and a bucket of water, he moves the bucket to the corner of the room and confidently states that he has reduced the situation to a solved problem.

An experimental physicist performs an experiment involving two cats, and an inclined tin roof. The two cats are very nearly identical: same sex, age, weight, breed, eye and hair color. The physicist places both cats on the roof at the same height and lets them both go at the same time. One of the cats falls off the roof first so obviously there is some difference between the two cats. What's the difference? One cat has a greater mew.

Why did the chicken cross the Mobius strip? To get to the same side.

Did you hear about the new exhibit at the physics department? They have a lepton conservatory.

There is this farmer who is having problems with his chickens. All of the sudden, they are all getting very sick and he doesn't know what is wrong with them. After trying all conventional means, he calls a biologist, a chemist, and a physicist to see if they can figure out what is wrong. So the biologist looks at the chickens, examines them a bit, and says he has no clue what could be wrong with them. Then the chemist takes some tests and makes some measurements, but he can't come to any conclusions either. So the physicist tries. He stands there and looks at the chickens for a long time without touching them or anything. Then all of the sudden he starts scribbling away in a notebook. Finally, after several gruesome calculations, he exclaims, "I've got it! But it only works for spherical chickens in a vacuum."

You know what they say about entropy? It's more than what it used to be.

Why won't Heisenberg's operators live in the suburbs? They don't commute.

All the famous scientists were sitting around heaven one day, contemplating the use of dice to make the universe go round. They realized that tomorrow was their annual "Great Scientist Convention" and again this year, Sir Isaac Newton was nowhere to be found. Almost certainly like last year he was out wandering the universe and would return just in time for the conference. All the great scientists convened and realized that one of them should go to the Pearly Gates to greet the great Sir Isaac upon his arrival. After much debate they settled on James Prescott Joule to stand watch for Sir Isaac's return for, as they all knew: Joule is a Newton-Meeter.

What's the difference between a mass spectrometer and a viola? You can tune a mass spectrometer.

Chapter 31

Think Soup!

"Mmm, Mmm Good."
- Campbell's Soup

June 7, 2003

One more week down! I now have nine radiation treatments (about 180 rads) and one chemo session behind me. This has been a better week. I'm recovering from the loss of appetite from the chemo treatment last week. This week consists of getting up, eating, getting up to the hospital to get irradiated, eating, eating, eating, and sleeping. I throw in a little woodworking, video games, cooking, piano playing, fly tying, yard work, laundry, and cleaning. Maybe I'll take up quilting.

Laura and I went to see Mama Mia in San Jose last weekend. It was a very nice night out with just the two of us. I will report that Mama Mia was loud (for us old folks) but a lot of fun. The lucky, elderly woman next to me was quite pleased that I didn't throw up on her – it was close.

We have started a new driving plan where a different friend from work drives me to treatment each day (day nine and I'm not out of friends yet!). It's working great. It gives me a chance to keep in touch, allows Laura to get in to work and takes a significant part of the stress out of our marriage – back seat driving. Yes – I'm a really bad back seat driver. When Laura is driving me on the freeway, all I can do is close my eyes and sleep. One would think that would work BUT... One day she caught me barking out directions with my eyes closed while dreaming about the traffic. And she thinks I have issues? Rob Hills takes me into treatment on Friday (after six different women in the previous seven days). The radiation technician asked me, "Run out of women?" My answer: "Hope not!"

Some good news (and bad news) – my white blood cell count was low but OK for ten days into the chemo (the normal low point).

Unfortunately, the warning is out that, if your white blood cell count is not low enough, they may up the dose next time. Wish I could rub that thermometer on the pants leg. Two more blood tests coming up this next week. I have successfully avoided fainting for each of the blood draws since returning from DC. It's close every time.

I have begun to feel some of the effects from the radiation. So far, swallowing is going well but my saliva glands are slowly being killed. This causes a whole host of problems starting with dry mouth and poor kissing technique. I'm discovering SOUP is a solution to many of my nutrition issues but you have to eat a lot of soup to gain weight. My neck is growing increasingly stiff (especially in the hours after the treatments). Another interesting side effect is ringing in the ears. Ever think about your cell phone ringing constantly? I'm thinking about asking for a tune change. I like Mozart.

I've also found some interesting information on the web. It turns out that those fun loving chemists (yeah the same group that brought us Cold Fusion) have a "molecule of the month" web site. Kind of like the swimsuit issue of sports illustrated for chemists. My chemo drug, cisplatin, made their calendar one month. It's officially called: cis-diamminedichloroplatinum(II). They even have a beautiful artist's rendition of cisplatin (shown below). The platinum is the pink one in the middle. They added on a couple of green Chlorines and two blue and white NH_3 groups. (Looks like something they are searching for in Iraq.) Also included in their molecule of the month list are such classics as ibuprofen, chlorophyll and sarin. And who says science isn't fun?

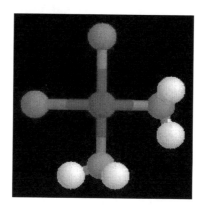

I've noticed a couple of interesting habits left over from my wine drinking days (hard to believe that two glasses a week will create "habits" – they were big glasses). I find myself swirling and sniffing the bouquet of my daily Ensure. That swirling action also perks up a nice hot cup of tea too. The nurse did stop me and ask why I was swirling my IV. I told her I was helping it breathe.

This week will be another good one! Four more radiation treatments will get me to the 1/3 mark. On Thursday (Our kids last day of school – both graduating – David moving on into Middle School and Sarah into High School), they put in my feeding tube. I'll miss the graduation festivities. Until next week, "Think soup!" I gotta keep swallowing.

Love, Mike

Chapter 32

Best Friends

*"We can stay up late, swapping manly stories,
and in the morning, I'm making waffles!"*
- Donkey, the Noble Steed, Shrek

Once upon a time in a far away land, there were two brothers named Mike and Uncle Ed that would come to really love each other some day (but not quite yet). Like most mornings when they were a kids (although not all that young during this story), Mike and Uncle Ed had relationship issues. On one particular morning, Uncle Ed was sleeping in and Mike just knew it was time for him to get up. What better way to get going in the morning than to rise to a beautiful viola serenade? So Mike broke out the instrument, rosined up the bow and quietly opened Uncle Ed's bedroom door and proceeded to wake him to the melodious tenor sounds of the viola (it turns out this is a felony in most states but not Ohio).

Mike must have misjudged Uncle Ed's mood somehow because he quickly took exception to Mike's humanitarian approach. Uncle Ed began objecting while still in bed but quickly got up and said something mean to his loving brother. Uncle Ed followed that with a gentle push. A couple of pushes later and Mike realized he had to put his finely crafted, French viola down to protect it from losing its tune (that's actually a good one but you need to be a Viola joke expert to get it). Mike retreated into the hall, placed his beloved instrument gently down on the dryer and proceeded to get shoved again by his irritated and ruthless sibling.

Well, Uncle Ed had crossed the line so Mike pushed him back. The push was a gentle one, like a gentle spring breeze in an alpine meadow, but it caught Uncle Ed off balance and he went backward down the hall like a defender under the basket trying to draw the charge. Uncle Ed chose to break his fall by colliding with the innocent dry wall. He hit the wall just right; hip and shoulder square between the studs. The dry wall was no match. Mike and Uncle Ed were stunned. Right there, in the middle of the hallway was a giant hole – 16 inches wide and a good 2.5 to 3 feet high. This was not good.

Luckily, Grandma was on the phone with a long-lost friend of hers. Her friend was one of those "perfect" friends with "perfect" kids and Grandma couldn't afford to yell at her own "perfect" children while on the phone. Grandma saw that her two "perfect" children were in trouble and slowly and quietly hung up. All Grandma could do was stare and say – "Just wait until your father gets home."

It was a long, torturous wait but Grandpa finally arrived. He was not at all happy but quickly had a vision. Over the next few weeks, Grandpa converted the hole in the wall into a built in mini-shelf to display Grandma's Hummel collection. From that day forward, that display shelf has been a topic of conversation, for both the collection and the origin of the shelf. To this day, Grandma's friend thinks Mike and Uncle Ed are perfect, and Mike and Uncle Ed have never fought again – and we never will!

Here's to my brother and best friend! (Good luck beating me in ping-pong.)

Chapter 33

Woody Allen?

"Be kinder than necessary because everyone you meet is fighting some kind of battle."
- Plato

June 15, 2003

Week three has come to an end! I now have thirteen radiation treatments behind me (with twenty two to go). This week was straightforward (except for Thursday). The radiation treatments continue to be routine – long drive with good friends, quick bolt down to the table (lasts about five minutes) and then they let me go. The side effects are just starting to build but are still very manageable. I successfully completed two blood draws this week with no significant threat of fainting (we'll get back to that). I'm still sleeping well, eating well (if it's wet) and I feel great!

On Monday, I met with Dr. Chinn (the radiation oncologist). I told him that I'd been recording and plotting my weight daily but had forgotten to print the plot and bring it with me. He told me that they were going to move me from gamma irradiation to high-energy electrons after week four (this will limit the dose to my spinal column to 40 Grays or 400 Rads). I began to ask about the electron energy (10MeV), the penetration depth (few cm), the number of irradiation angles (5) etc. His reply was – "when you bring the weight plot in next week, be sure it's plotted on a logarithmic scale." My response - "OK."

Do you think he's on to me?

Big news this week – Thursday was the placement of the feeding tube. Again, I don't need it yet but all predictors point to the need in the next few weeks. The placement was an outpatient procedure (although I was in the hospital from 7 am – 2:30 pm). I learned a few things:

(1) If at first your nurse can't get the IV in – Change nurses!

(2) Modern drugs are great things.

(3) Dr. Fredman (my Woody-Allen-movie GI Doctor) is from Illinois (I lost $100 on my Long Island bet).

So Dr. Fredman comes into the operating room and tells me that I'm now in good hands since he spent the day on Wednesday in a "heart restart training class." They always know just the right thing to say to help you relax.

They keep you awake for the procedure but they give you a drug that makes you forget what they did to you. The guy who thought of that is on my Christmas card list. They finally sent me home and told me not to look under the bandage. The next day, they sent us to the training class. Well, I struggled through the training class. First, they moved me to a chair with a back as I was showing outward signs of fainting at the sight of the tube. After the cold sweat broke, I realized that it's not all that bad. They sent me a month supply of formula (7 cans/day = 2100 calories). No need for a cork screw and, luckily, it's vanilla flavored. I caught myself swirling and enjoying the bouquet... Life's simple pleasures.

Last week, Milt Finger, a friend from work stopped by the house with a get-well card signed by Edward Teller. For those of you with a real life, Edward Teller is the father of the hydrogen bomb and the founder of both Lawrence Livermore Lab and the U.C. Davis, Department of Applied Science (where I got my Ph.D.). Dr. Teller is 95 years old. The hidden message – getting a card from him means I must really be in a world of hurt.

This week was a big week for the kids. David "graduated" from elementary school and Sarah "graduated" from middle school. For those of you with an aversion to the "brag and gag" style Christmas letter – PLEASE SKIP TO THE NEXT PARAGRAPH. If you are still reading, we are very proud of David and Sarah both. David has really developed into a good student and is really ready for the challenges of middle school. Sarah completed Middle School with a perfect 4.0 GPA over the three years. Sarah won the "All School" award (aka "nerd of the year") for the best overall student as voted on by the teachers. Although I missed the ceremony due to the surgery on Thursday, Laura videotaped it. Sarah accepted the award just above the shiny head of the bald guy in the foreground. I cried like a baby watching the tape. (I assume I cried because of the award and not at the thought of losing my hair).

So my hair has started to come out. So far, just the portion of the beard that is within the radiation field. That made the beard look like _____ (fill in the blank for yourself and email me your guess). So, I cut it all off. Laura says that shaving made it look like I lost twenty pounds.

This week will be another good one! I start Monday with an early irradiation and then it's off to my second chemo session. Judy Kammeraad tells me that the second chemo treatment will be easier – because – I now know what to expect. Well, I expect it to be worse. Worse but – tolerable. By the end of the week, I'll have passed the half way mark with 18 radiation treatments down. (Halfway through this phase of the cure.)

I'm still holding the wine in my collection. By the time I'm ready to drink it, I should have a few great bottles. The 2000 Bordeaux vintage is just beginning to hit the streets. This is the best vintage in the last 40 years but you have to hold them for 5-25 years. The big question: buy or pass? I should be buying.

The optimist in me says, "Buy it and hold. It'll get better with age." I want to be an optimist but I also want to drink the good stuff. This is indeed one of the world's great dilemmas.

Remember the difference between an optimist and a pessimist. A pessimist drinks his wine. An optimist is buried with a wine collection.

Love, Mike

Chapter 34

Little Mr. Williams

"Now this is not the end. It is not even the beginning of the end. But it is, perhaps, the end of the beginning."
  - Sir Winston Churchill

Once upon a time in a far away land there was a boy named Mike. Mike was just starting 7th grade. Believe it or not, this was the peak of his geek years. It was a broad "peak" – maybe more like a plateau. Those of you that know him now will be surprised to learn that he had significant social issues – yeah not just a geek thing but he had a severe stuttering problem. He had been through many years of speech therapy to no avail. Actually the speech therapy processes in elementary schools of suburban Cincinnati in the 1960s made the condition worse. The school nurse would come to Mike's classroom, interrupt the teacher and announce that it was time for Mike's speech therapy. As he left the room, his fellow classmates would laugh and tease him. Those classmates work for him now.

This entire process drove him further and further into his shell. He dreaded reading out loud, speaking in public or almost any talking in class. To survive, he learned a few tricks:

Trick number one: Lay low – pretend you really don't know the answer – the teachers will get tired of calling on you if they notice you at all.

Trick number two: Use word substitution – think ahead – if the word is going to be hard to say – think of another one and use it instead. Trick #2 works for casual conversation but is not nearly as effective reading Shakespeare in front of the class. "To exist or not to exist? That is the line of inquisition." It will also NOT work for words for which there is no substitute, like "Hello" when you answer the phone and... keep reading...

Trick number three: Get notes from your mother – get Mom to write a note to the teacher asking her to keep you in during recess… it's safer inside with the teacher. Playing chess does not require much speaking.

Well, along came day one of 7th grade. Mike was in Little Mr. Williams' social studies class. Little Mr. Williams was the smaller of the two Mr. Williams teachers at Anderson Middle School (hence his name). The taller is long forgotten by all who had him I'm certain. The shorter was cool, popular, and "famous." Everyone that was in Little Mr. Williams' class remembers him – of that too I am certain. In his spare time, he was an usher for the Cincinnati Reds in the blue seats behind home plate at Riverfront Stadium. Now remember, this is in the early 70s just as the Big Red Machine was in high gear. There was enormous excitement in Cincinnati about Pete Rose (Charlie Hustle), Johnny Bench (#5), Tony Perez ("baseball been berry, berry good to me"), Joe Morgan (the left elbow pump of our 5'4", base stealing, second baseman), Lee May (the Big Bopper from Birmingham), the spectacular center fielder César Geronimo (what a great name for a baseball player) and manager Sparky Anderson (even appeared on WKRP in Cincinnati). What a great time and place to be a baseball fan. Little Mr. Williams was an icon. He had bright red hair and was certainly the most popular teacher in the school. Mike was going to have him for social studies – life was looking up!

Back to day one – all students had assigned seats, in alphabetical order. Mike was a "C" placing him in the back of the room in the first row. At the beginning of class, each student was asked to stand, in order, state their name and tell the class something fun they did on their summer vacation. Simple right? Trick number one will not work - he was going to get Mike when it was his turn. Trick number 2? Well, "Carter" is a difficult name. It starts with a difficult to pronounce hard consonant and word substitution is not appropriate – it is Mike's last name. It was finally Mike's turn. He stood up in the back corner of a classroom full of kids he knows and in front of the coolest teacher he had ever seen and said. "My name is Mike C… C… C… C… C… C… Mike C… C… C… C… C… C… C…"

Little Mr. Williams interrupted when it became clear Mike was struggling just to say his name and said, "Don't throw up on us or something!"

The class erupted in laughter. With the tension broken, Mike blurted out "Mike Carter" followed by a quick, lame summer story and sat down. (Too bad I was too old for trick three).

Little Mr. Williams turned out to be the coolest teacher ever but - what a start.

I saw Little Mr. Williams just a few years ago at Skyline Chili in Mt. Washington, Ohio. He hadn't changed a bit except maybe a little less red hair. I had lots of things I wanted to tell him including the tale above, but I thought he might not understand the positive nature of the story. He's still working the Reds – no more Big Red Machine, no more blue seats, no more Riverfront Stadium. He didn't recognize me but I didn't stutter. Like King George, I finally got over my stuttering for the most part in high school. Someone finally realized that I didn't stutter in music, math, or science classes. Interesting. It was all about confidence.

To this day, the people closest to me (those that have "seen me naked") can tell when I'm lying, stretching the truth, or just not confident in my story line... I stutter.

Chapter 35

Low on Hotel Soap

"I have second thoughts. Maybe God is malicious."
- Albert Einstein

June 21, 2003

Week four brought some new and interesting issues to the Carter household. I now have 18 radiation treatments behind me (18/35) so I'm just over half way done with stage II of the tour de head and neck cancer. (Stage 1 = diagnosis and surgeries, stage II = chemo/radiation, stage III = chemo just for the fun of it, stage IV = the remainder of my life).

Week four of stage II began with a radiation treatment early Monday morning. I brought in my weight plot charted on a logarithmic plot and the doctor called me a smart ass (success at last!). It is much easier to hold your weight on a logarithmic plot.

Radiation was followed by five hours sitting in the chemo chair. Chemotherapy day one is not that big a deal, just sitting in the chair for six hours while they run water and poison through your system. I was joined in the festivities (the sitting not the poison) by my wife, my mother, and my friend Ellen Tarwater. Dr. Russin told us on Monday that I wouldn't lose my hair – well – come the end of the week, we think it's falling out. Those Doctor predictions are good as gold.

Day two brought some new adventures (like nausea and vomiting). This drags you into day three (the nap day). Day four should be the day you begin to exit out of the thrills but some battles with the phlegm gods got the best of me.

Friday came and I began to feel human again (just barely). This recovery was slower than the last one but I'm still holding my own on the log scale.

I'm still looking for volunteers to shave their heads in sympathy. Any other sympathy gestures will be welcome with the most spectacular earning a special award of distinction (you'll like it when I come up with it).

Significant trauma has struck the Carter household. With all the traveling I have done over the past few years, I have absconded with numerous hotel soaps and shampoos. Well, we're running low and I'm scared. I don't think I can shower without Marriott shampoo. I need help! Donations are desperately needed. (Towels, sheets and pillowcases are still in abundant supply).

I had some visitors from the east on Saturday. Tony, Ralph (and his five kids), and Maureen and David all stopped by. We feel like the prime tourist spot in California. Word of the considerable joy obtained from spending time with me and my box of Kleenex has not yet spread to the east (as is evidenced by continued visits).

Research results are out – Kleenex beat Scotties in rigorous series of tests. Due to the advanced, pre-deployment mechanism implemented by Kleenex in the mid 70's, Kleenex are ultimately deployed from their container in a fraction of the time required for alternate brands such as Scotties. While this advantage is considered minimal by many researchers, urgency and the cloak of darkness can often lead to situations were even a few milliseconds can make the difference between system-level success or failure. These results should be considered final in our household.

And this just in: Campbell's' Chicken and Stars Soup is in fact a "fun favorite" as described on the label. Watch out – there are some big hunks of pasta in that soup.

Love and thanks for all the support. I continue to count on it!

Mike

Chapter 36

Uncle Edie

"Not that there's anything wrong with that."
- Jerry Seinfeld

Once upon a time in a far away land there was a boy named Uncle Ed. Uncle Ed had Little Mr. Williams for both English and History class in the 7th grade at Anderson Middle School. Little Mr. Williams ran his classes like a competition. This year he had decided to break the class into two teams, the Girls and the Boys. Unfortunately for Uncle Ed, there were four more boys than girls in the English class. Little Mr. Williams announced that there would be a competition and "since everyone knows the girls are dumber than the boys, the two dumbest boys would join the girls' team for the year where they belong." Much to Uncle Ed's dismay, the competition was a spelling bee; not Uncle Ed's strongest suit. Uncle Ed and Jeff Block were the first two boys eliminated and immediately and permanently became known as Edie and Jenny. It was announced that hereafter, in Mr. Williams Classes (English and History) Uncle Ed was to be considered a girl and called Edie! In general this turned out to be a bonus as in reality 7th grade girls are way smarter than 7th grade boys and, due to this sexual misidentification, Edie's grades improved significantly.

In history class, Edie found herself/himself on more favorable turf. One of the competitions was World and Ohio geography. During the competition, two students would stand at the front of the class and Little Mr. Williams would shout out a country in Africa. The first student to locate that country on a map would win and advance to the next competitor. Well, Edie was a whiz at maps and could roll through the competition. Mr. Williams would shout to the boys in the class "For GOD'S SAKE, you are being beaten by a girl!" This healthy competition and sexual identity crisis made Edie the woman/man he is today. (Edie is still a world-class bad speler)

Little Mr. Williams would also run the occasional "free A" competition. The class was asked if they wanted to participate and "bet" a free A on the Kentucky Derby. A Win was a free A, Place was a free B, Show was a free C, all others were free F's. It was 1972 and Edie pulled a horse's name out of the hat. Aunt/Uncle Edie drew Secretariat – the rest is history. Aunt/Uncle Edie got an "A" in the class (along with most of the other girls).

Chapter 37

Drinking and Politics

"Help! Help! I'm being repressed!"
- Dennis, Monty Python and the Holy Grail

June 28, 2003

Week five has come and gone! 23 of 35 radiation treatments are behind me! And this was a much better week than last. The drag from the chemo last week has lifted and the old positive attitude has returned. I just can't describe how dreadful that chemo is. It almost sucks the will to live from you. But this week brought heat to California (107 was the high on Wednesday) and my appetite is back. The doctors, nurses and technicians kept telling me this week would be bad but I missed something – I feel GREAT!

Eating, while a challenge, has gotten better. I'm still using the feeding tube to be sure my weight is up. It is also good patience practice (it's not fast). I have also developed some slow eating habits. This does NOT mean I will emerge a patient person – I'll just be refining my "European eating skills." I have also learned to be quick on the Kleenex draw. I can pull and wipe a Kleenex as fast as the French can wave a white flag. (This comment is not intended to influence the wine-buying public. As my friend Richard says "I separate my politics from my wine drinking.")

My big battle continues to be with the phlegm gods, Fred and Ethyl. I figure, if they are going to move in with you, you might as well name them and give them personalities. They might be guests for a long time so I'd better know how to deal with them.

The radiation treatments appear to be going well (I have no unexcused absences and no tardies). They started me on a 10MeV electron diet this week (to limit the dose to the spinal column). I guess 400 Rads is about the limit the spinal cord can take. The electrons deposit their energy in the first few cm of the neck (where it's needed) and allow them to continue to irradiate the tissue and protect the spine. Getting hit with 10MeV reminds me of the good old days in the lab with David Whelan. Dave got hit with everything! He's much better suited for office work. You know, if we did this stuff at work (hit someone with 400 Rads, 10MeV electrons or 6 MeV Gammas) they would cancel the UC contract.

On Thursday, the radiation therapist caught me snoring on the table. That mask must not be so bad after all. This week they will begin to taper off on the irradiation (a sign that it is coming to an end). The doc says he will run me through the MRI in Mid July to see if any of this is working. I can't wait! Better leave Fred and Ethel at home for that hour in the tube. Fred and Ethyl are claustrophobic. The Doctor has not yet discussed the details of the follow-up chemo with us. His last comment was "We'll try to get you through it." I hope they know what they are doing.

This week brought a personal, hand signed note from Dick Cheney. He and Lynne are counting on me to hold on long enough to vote Republican in the 2004 presidential election. I promised to vote absentee if I have to (I might have to register in Chicago where you can vote twice). Carol K – if you were behind this – THANKS!

Sarah got her summer reading assignment for honors English (To Kill a Mockingbird and The Chosen). I drafted a fake letter from the school with a six book reading assignment including War and Peace and a warning about six weeks of summer school in 2004. She was not amused. Not everyone thinks I'm funny.

We went to see Finding Nemo. I had some sleep deprivation issues and missed "Losing Nemo" at or near the beginning. I did wake up before they found him but I think I missed the point of the movie. Didn't even cry when they finally got together.

Only four days of treatment this coming week (Cancer doesn't grow on the weekends or Federal holidays). I'll get in some naps here and there but I expect to be feeling quite good. Next Chemo is on July 7th Keep the email coming! I enjoy the notes. Thanks for all the support. I continue to count on it!

Love, Mike

Chapter 38

Watch Out

"Is there someone else up there we could talk to?"
- Sir Galahad

"I think I cold pull through, sir"
- Concorde, Monty Python and the Holy Grail

In case the point is not clear, visitors are very welcome and important in the Carter household. Even while suffering the side effects of radiation treatments and chemotherapy, the pick-me-up is stimulating and motivating. It gives renewed hope, purpose and determination in the quest to get this behind me. It also reminds me of the down side of failure.

One of the challenges in accepting visitors is expectation management. They must also "learn" to accept you as you are. Cleaning the house or bathing and dressing must be considered optional. We're not trying to impress anyone just as they are not trying to impress us (for the most part).

One set of unmentionable visitors, lets call them Bill and Sally to preserve their secret identities, stopped in to visit one day. I knew Sally very well from a substantive work relationship and I had met Sally's husband (Bill) on a few occasions. Laura didn't know either of them but had heard many a Sally story. They were a very interesting couple – both PhDs in some field of science. Sally was bright and energetic. Bill was mature, intelligent, quiet, good-looking and very British (with a great accent). I swear, the Brits sound smarter than they are with their big vocabularies and fancy accents. I also think their relative formality in their interactions makes them seem more thoughtful than the bold, brash, in-your-face American style (especially during the Bush administration). I will admit to a few cringes watching Tony Blair and George Bush at a joint press conference.

Our visit with "Bill and Sally" went as usual. I sat on the couch in my pajamas with my feeding tube rolled and tucked neatly under my shirt trying to be as inconspicuous as possible. Laura sat by my side holding my hand and doing her best to be a social butterfly (though with clipped wings). These interactions were hard on her for many reasons. A stranger traveling across the country to visit her sick husband was well outside her comfort zone. She was generally quiet. The conversation centered on work as it most often does with a few "sick stories" mixed in. Bill displayed the British wit they are known for and for some reason, it must have been the lighting and the fancy accent, Bill took on a faint resemblance to Hugh Grant or Colin Firth. He was a pretty cool guy.

After the hour and a half visit, Bill and Sally made their way on to the next destination in life (hopefully not another sick friend) and Laura and I returned to the comfort of our kitchen. I asked Laura what she thought of Bill and Sally. Her response was priceless: "If you don't make it, I'm going after Bill."

I guess I need to make it (and maybe work on my accent).

Chapter 39

Kids

"Dad, you're not funny."
- Sarah Carter

July 6, 2003

Well, we're making progress. I've completed week six of the radiation treatments (27 treatments down, eight to go). In fact, this was kind of a turn-the-corner week. They have begun to back off on the daily dose (down from five exposures per day to only 3). They have also started to give me radiation burns. Some of it is interesting physics. My neck, face and chest are all "sun burnt" but even though they don't irradiate me from behind, so is my back. Those gamma rays go right through you. I'm burned on the inside too – really fun way to celebrate the 4th of July.

We went to the Clower's for the 4th of July (as always). I had been watching the food network on TV and had seen a recipe for beer can chicken. It involves slow cooking a chicken while it sits on a half-full beer can (and I thought I had it rough). I also made my mother-in-law's cinnamon rolls (for the kids) and we had a great time. This year we embarrassed the kids by naming all the different fireworks after famous galactic nebula. There is nothing like watching fireworks with a geek.

Boy have I discovered a whole world out there. Not only is there the Food Network but also, the Golf Channel, OLN (televises the entire Tour d' France), the Bowling Channel and the Quilting Channel. Will the action in the Carter household ever cease? I'll go satellite when the woodworking channel hits the air.

I'm continuing to eat through this ordeal. Again, it really helps if the food is wet. I have discovered that Fred and Ethyl are not big Jell-O fans. As such, it's not unusual to eat a cup of Jell-O at 2, 4 and 6 am. If anyone else has any pointers, I'm listening. My voice is starting to become weak (much to the joy of many of my family members). I'm hoping to emerge from this summer vacation with a little more patience and some better listening skills.

For fun this week, I hosted the Q-Division administrators meeting. The two highlights there were a talk on the Department of Homeland Security and a detailed discussion of lingerie modeling (it's a long story but suffice it to say, I was not a threat).

I continue to enjoy the company of my friends who generously volunteer to drive me to radiation treatments every day. They have no idea how much they are saving me on lawyer fees. If the doctors figured in the "driving with the wife" risk to my five-year survival, my odds would be skyrocketing - downward.

The doctors and nurses continue to tell me how well I'm doing. Laura keeps asking me if I'm telling them the truth. I have felt pretty good this week (a little dragging over the weekend as the sore throat and "sunburn" builds). The oncology office called on the 4th and informed me that my white blood cell count was too low to proceed with the chemo on Monday – so – go take another blood test – maybe it will go up. I immediately started to drag (classic psycho symptoms). We'll know Monday morning if they will pump in the poison or not. I just want to get it over with.

A few miscellaneous complaints:

1) I have not lost my hair yet – all that money on hats.

2) Fred and Ethyl need to visit Lucy and Ricky for one night.

3) My printer doesn't work – I hate printers!

4) I wish my kids thought I was funny – like they used to.

Here's to a good week. I'm hoping they get the chemo go ahead and I can complete Phase II of this four-ring circus on time!

Thanks for support. I look forward to your emails. Warning! Our email address has changed. We're victims of another corporate takeover – we should get the golf channel for free!

Love, Mike

Chapter 40

The Dead Fish

"Get your facts first, then you can distort them as you please."
         - Mark Twain

Once upon a time there was a boy named Al. One evening Al and his friends, Mike, Lou, and Eric, decided to go fishing. They decided to go to RonJo lake. RonJo was a "pay lake" not too far from their house where it cost money to fish but they were guaranteed to catch fish. The plan was to fish all night, catch lots of fish, and take them home to Al's Mom to cook. They got to the lake just before dark and fished for an hour or so without even a single bite. Mike was getting bored and decided they *all* need some cokes and chips. Mike put another dough ball on his fishing line and casted it as far into the lake as he could. He put his pole down and he and Eric got in the car and headed to the closest mini-market.

While Mike and Eric were out on their humanitarian mission to bring food and drink to all their fishing friends, Al searched the edge of the lake looking for the biggest dead fish he could find. Al found a huge catfish and hatched a plan. Al pulled Mike's line in hooked the dead fish in the mouth and casted it back into the lake. Unfortunately, the fish floated on the surface – not the plan. Al reeled it back in and stuffed the fish's mouth with rocks. He then casted the fish back out into the lake and it sank to the bottom. Al then returned the rod to the same position Mike had left it.

Mike and Eric returned with enough coke and chips to feed the Donner Party. Mike went for his rod to see if he had caught anything while he was gone. He began to reel and said, "I think I caught one"

"It's a big one."

"It's really fighting!"

As the fighting monster got closer to shore something didn't seem quite right.

"Hey, I think it's dead" Mike uttered as he landed the giant catfish.

Looking more closely, Mike reportedly said, "No wonder it's dead, it's been eating rocks!"

[The official version ends differently with Mike *actually* saying "Who put rocks in this fish's mouth Al?" – the pen of history is mine and my self-esteem is intact!]

Chapter 41

Lawn Darts

"If you're going through hell, keep going."
- Sir Winston Churchill

July 13, 2003

We were right about this week (we hope). This was the toughest week to date. Almost done with stage II now. All three chemos are behind me (barely) and I have only three more radiation treatments to go. But it was almost not to be...

It all started on Monday morning with a phone call to the house (after we had left) telling us our chemotherapy session had been canceled due to my white blood cell count being very low. When we arrived at the hospital (having missed the call) they decided to draw more blood and see if they could proceed. In the meantime, the doctor called in sick himself (I bet I felt worse than he did). Somehow, even though my count was not up and the doctor was not in, they decided to proceed. So we started the fluid; got the anti-nausea drugs in, worked the kidneys, and dumped in the poison.

We then proceeded to run up to the radiation clinic where, they too had decided to cancel the treatment due to the low white blood cell count. After some confusion about why the chemotherapy had proceeded (this time discussing it with a doctor), they decided if I could handle the chemotherapy, I could handle the radiation so – zap away. This odd decision-making process saved me at least three or four days and prevented a gap in the radiation treatment cycle. (Gaps in radiation do not read well in the clinical trials).

My orders were simple – stay clear of infections, people, dirt, grime, germs, soft cheeses, leftovers, fresh vegetables, sushi, raw shellfish, etc... This was relatively easy – all I wanted to do was sleep all week. So I slept. I averaged four to five naps per day (two to three hours each) leaving all of ten or fifteen minutes to get dirty. They also started me on daily injections of Neupogen to get my count up. (This ended on Thursday when my counts shot up out of range on the high side)

The week went by relatively quickly (sleeping will do that). I found that watching Lance Armstrong on the "Lance Armstrong network" was inspirational. Watching Lance helped me cut my nap times by a few minutes each day. I have no idea how he does it.

They have continued to back off on the daily radiation dose (down from five exposures per day to only two). The radiation burns are not as bad as I expected. Face it, radiation is your friend! I'm completely done with the electrons and the gamma ray fields are getting smaller and smaller as they zoom in on the highest dose areas. You read about getting extremely tired toward the end of the radiation ordeal. Well, I'm too tired to read. Even Harry Potter is on hold.

Some of the side effects are worse than others. Fred and Ethel are still with me (any side effect with a nickname is not a good one). Each successive chemotherapy seems to take a little longer to recover from. Chemotherapy causes ringing in the ears and sensitivity to noise. It also seems to cause neuropathy (a general numbness which one might think could be a good thing).

I continue to have trouble sustaining my weight the week after chemo. I point out that I've lost almost twenty-five pounds since April. Laura notes that I've put on fifteen pounds since our wedding. (You do NOT want to see those pictures).

This week will bring the radiation to a close and will certainly stimulate some celebration. They say it takes a week or more to get the energy back after the radiation treatments end. I'm ready.

Until next week, thanks to all for the support. Feel free to send emails – I look forward to them. We'll be watching the British Open, the Tour d' France and the World Championship of Lawn Darts this week.

Love, Mike

Chapter 42

After the Loving

"If only I had known, I should have become a watch maker."
- Albert Einstein

In about 1995 I had the opportunity to take my father and brother, Ed, on a tour of the Nevada Test Site. This was after the end of the nuclear test program and the test site had become a much quieter place. We were working on buried land mine detection technologies and had established a buried object test site in Yucca Flats simulating the physics of detection of buried mines in desert environments. One of my closest friends and "cohorts in crime," David Fields, and I were both staying in Las Vegas the night before the tour so we had two rooms reserved. Our plan was to share a room and let my Dad and my brother stay in the other.

The story starts with Dave Fields arriving in Las Vegas before me, Dad and Ed (by a few hours) and attempting to check into the hotel. Dave was notorious about money (never having any cash on him) and his credit card (which he had failed to pay the bill on time) was once again rejected by the hotel. You know what they say – "what happens in Vegas, stays in Vegas" but only if your credit card clears. By the time we arrived, Dave's room with two beds had been given away to someone with a higher credit score. The only unreserved rooms remaining were outfitted with single, queen-sized beds. I checked into my room (two beds – one for Dad, one for Ed) and also used my credit card to get a room for Dave and me; a room with one queen sized bed was all they had left. We asked for a rollaway to be moved in and they agreed. We were not sleeping together – you have to draw the line somewhere! We quickly went off to dinner and a run at the casinos. It was time to eat and put my $20 at risk. Dave had no intention of putting anything other than my money at risk.

When we returned to the room, it was getting late. We had planned a very early start the next morning (5am departure from Vegas) to be sure we had plenty of time to tour the Test Site.

Walking into the room about midnight, we saw that the rollaway bed was folded up in the entryway and had not been made up. We both took one look at the Queen-sized bed, and another at the rollaway. We looked at each other and agreed, "You're not going to touch me are you?" We would leave the rollaway alone and just get to sleep – together in a queen-sized bed. What happens in Vegas, stays in Vegas.

I went in to brush my teeth and change my clothes. Dave followed when I was done. As he was brushing his teeth, I turned on the radio and found Engelbert Humperdinck singing, "After the Loving, I'm still in love with you." I turned up the radio and started singing along. The next thing I knew, Dave was unfolding the rollaway, putting on the sheets and sleeping by himself! So was I.

The next day, the four of us were off to the Nevada Test Site. Our first stop was the old above-ground nuclear testing area on Frenchman Flat. There are some very interesting nuclear ruins. Blasted walls, bunkers, hangers, bridges, and railroad tracks litter the landscape. There are signs warning visitors to not touch any metal objects, as they may be radioactive. My Dad had the bad habit of collecting a souvenir from places he had been (e.g. a rock from the top of Pikes Peak). Dad picked up a big (1&1/2" diameter) bolt with a huge rusty nut. I warned him that it was probably radioactive (since it was near ground zero of a half-dozen nuclear explosions) and I could get in a lot of trouble if he was caught with it. He reluctantly and grudgingly put the nut and bolt back, made some smart remark, and we continued the tour. I recall something like, "A little radiation never hurt anybody." He was, in fact, a world-renowned expert on such science (and a banker in Cincinnati).

We had a great day visiting the Sedan Crater, Rainier Mesa, Piute Mesa overlooking Area 51, the BREN Tower and all the big sights of NTS. Just after we exited the gate at Mercury, Dad pulled the nut and bolt out of his pocket and said, "See, you didn't get caught." He was such a pain!

Two years later, Dad was diagnosed with pancreatic cancer and died six weeks after the diagnosis. Ed and I were searching his belongings for his Masonic Lodge sash for the funeral service. Searching through his underwear drawer, we found that big, old, rusty, (radioactive) nut and bolt. We decided to put the nut and bolt in the casket with Dad so if they ever needed to find him they could use either a metal detector or a Geiger counter.

Chapter 43

Sorry

"Just raise your hand if you need help."
- John Doe – Radiation Dose Enhancement Specialist

July 20, 2003

Phase II is officially over. We completed the last radiation treatment on July 16th (right on schedule) and I am officially on "vacation" from the doctors! But it was not without it's own special challenges.

As Mr. Rogers would say, Monday was a "special day in the neighborhood." I had accepted much praise from the radiation technicians (Radiological Dose Enhancement Specialists as they should be called in this Politically Correct world). I took the opportunity on Monday to throw up on them – yeah well, it's not as easy to behave as the emails might lead you to believe. I never thought they could move so fast. Twenty minutes later, they bolted me back to the table and got even. Tuesday was uneventful except I noticed they were all keeping their distance. The hugs and kisses from the day before were replaced by a bucket resting on my lap.

Tuesday night was a good one. Just as I'm getting emotionally ready to close the radiation treatments on Wednesday, the Oncology department calls (at 8:30 pm) asking about the next surgical procedure (August 8). They want to know if the doctor has told me what they are planning to do or not. Of course, they don't know and the doctor is not there at 8:00 pm – (oncologists work 9-5). They just take all the fun out of having a good day. By the way – they are planning to install a PICC line to administer the drugs in Phase III.

Wednesday was a day for celebration. Finally, the last of 35 radiation treatments is approaching. (I brought in a peace offering – homemade toffee from Aunt Ruth's secret recipe). I had pulled it off with limited pain and suffering. The sunburn was deep but no real blistering or significant peeling. I calculated a total of 2540 seconds of 6 MeV gamma ray beam time (42 minutes) plus about 800 seconds of 10 MeV electrons (only about 13 minutes). We went through about ten different shielding geometries and I had more than twenty x-rays. All this happened while driving more than 3,000 miles with 18 different drivers (including myself – I drove once).

We get home from our last treatment and sitting in the driveway is the FedEx truck. I'm thinking – YEAH! Gifts and prizes. I asked for whatever was behind door number three and sure enough – A giant box from Jack Foreman (friend from DC). Inside the box: four bags of candy – clearly labeled "for Sarah and David" and two coffee cans full of Marriott Hotel soap and shampoo! I'm back in business.

So along came Thursday. I'm washing my hair the good, old-fashioned way – with free shampoo. Free shampoo seems to lather better. All cleaned up and nowhere to go… I'm bored (obviously). I'm expecting to feel better already. I'm disappointed. Emotional letdowns are so predictable and yet, so unavoidable. You'd think we would be smarter than that… maybe I'll break into the free soap.

A simple ethical question: What do you do when the disability insurance lady calls to "see how you are doing"? Do you act really sick – coughing, spitting, nausea, weakness etc. or do you suck it up and pretend like you can't wait to get back to work? I'm torn. The truth is somewhere in between but the insurance company has no category for "wants to work but still too sick to be effective."

The doctors are planning some follow up scans (MRI, CAT) in about 6-8 weeks. As Judy has told me, cancer patients learn about patience. No reason to do a scan sooner as the radiation leaves significant tissue damage that is in the process of healing. This healing tissue can easily be confused with active tumor and lead to false readings. The scans don't really change the treatment strategy they just give the doctors and patients a taste of the soup half way through. If it tastes bad, they just keep simmering. If it tastes good, they keep simmering. The only difference – you might schedule that cruise a little sooner and upgrade the cabin.

The follow-up plan:

1) Get Lance to hold his lead all the way to Paris.

2) Begin phase three – three chemotherapy treatments (cisplatin and 5-FU) spaced four weeks apart beginning August 11.

3) Get some scans done (sometime in late August or early September).

4) Get feeling better! – I'm well on the way to that one already.

5) Schedule that cruise – later – no upgrade.

Love, Mike

Chapter 44

For the Record, I've been Near Death Before

"Oh the humanity!"
- Les Nessman, WKRP in Cincinnati

Once upon a time in a far away land there were two boys named Mike and Ed. They lived a few miles south of a quiet village named Madeira. The name Madeira is from the old Indian Hill word meaning – "poor people, come visit at your own risk." Madeira, Ohio was one of those places where the rich people live. Mike and Ed's planned transit through Madeira was facilitated by the one mistake a commoner made years before – they put a road through. Now, mind you, this road had a questionable safety record but that would turn out to play a role in the dropped charges at the end of the day.

Mike and Ed had a hard working, normally loving mother who was slaving away at the near-by Milford School District Board of Education offices. Their Mom must have been under a lot of stress, because apparently, it didn't sound like a death sentence to allow her two darling children into a car with a stick shift and no seat belts, driven by her baby sister (the boys' beloved Aunt Sara) with very limited driving experience. (Checking back on the records, Mike and Ed's parents purchased life insurance policies for their two boys right about this same time – this could have had a mind-numbing effect on their normally good parental judgment. In a possible conspiracy angle, they named *themselves* the beneficiaries – raises the blades of grass on the back of my grassy knoll).

Aunt Sara had decided to take Mike and Ed to see Uncle Leonard that afternoon. On the way home, Aunt Sara had to exit Madeira by driving up the dreaded Madeira Hill in the stick shift. This was not an ordinary stick shift but a blue, 1960 Chevrolet Corvair. Many a niece or nephew has been unexpectedly maimed, killed, scarred for life, or worse in the vehicle Ralph Nader would come to describe as "unsafe at any speed." Aunt Sara was about to prove

Ralph right. We thought of it as a "blue death trap with a stick shift."

Before I recount the dreaded event, let me grab a few Kleenex just in case the psychological trauma becomes too much for me again. Aunt Sara pulled halfway up the hill and the traffic light ahead turned red. Aunt Sara and her innocent passengers were stuck behind a rich lady right on the steep part of the slope. Another rich lady with questionable judgment pulled up right behind them.

Why the rich-woman-with-a-death-wish pulled up so close to rear bumper of the Nadar death trap is beyond me. She should have known that stopping anywhere within about fifty feet of Aunt Sara was going to cause stress in the beautiful, intelligent, popular, rhombus-loving, varsity cheerleading Aunt (for the record, she was not in uniform). When the light turned green all hell broke loose. The actual events are too blurred to be completely accurate but the blue Corvair bumped the car in front at least once and the car behind them about a half dozen times. Oh the Humanity! Screams pierced the paper-thin boundaries of the blue death trap. It seemed like time and clutch skills collided and then, only God knows what happened.

Aunt Sara's Corvair finally leapt from the bumper of the rich lady's car behind them and sped off. The poor frightened, unbelted, scared-for-life, children in the back seat were left with only two things – shaken confidence in Aunt Sara's driving abilities at the tender age of 16 years and 2 months and a story that is like a fine wine – it will last many decades, getting better and better as time goes by.

Chapter 45

No Nothing

*"Death is very likely the single best invention of life,
it is life's change agent."*
- Steve Jobs

July 27, 2003

This will be a tough update to write so I'll keep it short. Not a single thing happened this week on the medical front. No doctors, no nurses, no blood, no guts, no nausea. It was a good week – every day, I felt noticeably better. In general they are small increments but the trend is in the right direction. All in all, I had a much better week than Uday, Qusay and Governor Gray Davis.

We were blessed with family visitors this week. My mother is still here helping nurse me back to health. She heads back to her life in Cincinnati on Wednesday. Mom was joined by my brother (Ed), sister-in-law (Joan) and their two kids, Matt and Ellen. They all stayed with our great friends, Curtis and Ellen Clower. They head for home in Minneapolis on Thursday.

Our niece, Amy, stopped in the bay area for the weekend and stayed with us. The big challenge is meals. First we have me – preferring to eat foods that are wet; our son - cereal, pizza, peanut butter sandwiches (no jelly) and junk food; Laura – no veggies; Amy – veggies only; plus all the company. It was not unusual to fix 5-6 different meals at a time. This dysfunction can only last a short time.

I'm starting to feel good enough to get some exercise (walking). I am eating much better and actually put on a few pounds this week. I figure I'm at a great weight right here (if I were running 7 minute miles). My secondary goal over the next year is to gain three pounds and shave 4 minutes off my time. The primary goal remains the same and should be obvious to even the casual observer – stay married! Makes the seven-minute mile looks easy...

Still exploring the overnight entertainment options. I've been looking for the 3am eBay special on Grape Jell-O. Somehow I need to exchange my two-hour afternoon nap and my two-hour overnight anti-nap. As my GI doctor might say, "this too shall pass."

Struggled with Kaiser some this week trying to find additional bandages to help hold my feeding tube in place. They gave me three at the training class and now claim no knowledge of anything to do with them. It's like Hillary and the Rose Hill Law Firm records (sorry to mix medicine and politics). After discussions with a half dozen "helpers" at Kaiser, I've decided it's a conspiracy led by the mental health professionals – they are trying to drive me crazy! I'll just use that Homeland Security-approved duct tape – comes off with the first layer of skin.

Not much to report coming up this week. Our kids travel to Minnesota with my brother's family for a week in Minneapolis and a week at summer camp. I will be childless for the first time in 14 years. Laura will still have me to deal with. I miss them already and they aren't even gone yet. Laura and I will have no idea what to do.

We expect no interactions with the medical professionals this week – unless their bandage conspiracy matures. Electroshock could be good for me – I'll try to find a clinical trial to join.

Until next week – keep those emails pouring in (the river has shrunk to a small stream). I miss you all!

Love, Mike

Chapter 46

Casper

"There's a sucker born every minute."
  - P.T. Barnum

Once upon a time, in a far away land, there were two boys named Mike and Ed. They were just little guys (about 4 & 6 years old). Every Sunday morning in Cincinnati there was a TV show they really liked: The Skipper Ryle Show. Skipper Ryle played cartoons and had a live studio audience (kids and parents) to cheer for him and play a few cool games. The show was filmed in a studio somewhere in downtown Cincinnati, probably WCPO Channel 9 studios. One Sunday morning, Mike and Ed decided to go and be members of the studio audience.

One of the "cool" games they played was a "swap meet" where each kid would bring a toy to trade with the other kids. Mike took his highly coveted "Casper the Friendly Ghost" board game, knowing he could trade it for something even more cool. The trading game worked by calling kids up to the front (during the running of the cartoons) and the kid called up would get to pick a kid in the audience to trade with. Mike waved his Casper game like a French surrender flag. Time after time, no one picked him. Didn't they know how cool Casper was? To be sure no child went home unhappy, they also gave each kid a goodie bag with candy, some cheap toys (maybe a yoyo or a plastic spinning top), a toothbrush and toothpaste (it was probably sponsored by Procter and Gamble). Well, as the end of the show rolled around, Mike was holding his goodie bag and that darn "Casper the Friendly Ghost" game. He really didn't want to go back home humiliated with the same toy he had come with. What's a kid to do?

Well, Mike traded his Casper game to the kid behind him for a tube of toothpaste.

Let the humiliation begin.

Chapter 47

Less than Nothing

"Nothin from Nothin leaves Nothin."
- The Commodores on Math

August 3, 2003

Even less happened this week than last. Not even a phone call from the medical establishment. Have they forgotten about me? They know that I'm getting "back to normal" and they are planning a counter attack. I'll beat them in the end.

This week saw some major accomplishments: my first hamburger since April, my first steak, and my first realization that I'm about through with this feeding tube. OK, the hamburger was only 2/3 eaten before I gave up – I figure it's like one of those speed chess games. If after twenty minutes, you haven't figured it out – it's time to quit. OK, the steak was the fatty corner of a grilled rib eye but – I ate half of it! These "normal" foods are still a struggle but I'm dangerous with a can of soup. I'm really out on the limb tonight – trying Lime Jell-O instead of Grape – wish me luck.

Our company is back home now. Mom returned to Cincinnati on Wednesday after a seven-week stay. I'm sure she's a lot happier to get home than we are to lose her. She was a bigger help than she knows. My brother and his family returned to Minneapolis on Thursday – and they took our kids with them. That's right – Laura and I are home alone. This sounds way better than it is. It's hard to believe how much we rely on the kids. Without them – there is nothing to talk about, no one to yell at, no one to praise, no one to look at except each other. When they go off to college, we'll be lost! They've been gone now for three days and I'm not sure I'll make it the full two weeks.

My brother Ed and I had an interesting adventure trying to run a new sprinkler line under the walkway. It turns out – there are already some sprinkler lines (including the main feed line) there in the way. We realized this when we broke through them. It was kind of like going to Yellowstone and witnessing Old Faithful. Lucky for me, the repair involved blind PVC patching at arms length, in the mud, under the walkway. The advantages of the feeding tube were obvious – "I can't lay on my stomach and do that – it's too dangerous for me – you'll have to do it Ed." OK – I'll keep the feeding tube a while longer.

Laura and I went up to a friend's cabin in the Sierras on Friday night. It was a beautiful evening (which we needed after getting caught in an hour-long traffic jam not twenty minutes out of Livermore). We were awoken in the middle of the night by a spectacular mountain thunderstorm (and a cabin without power). It rained all morning the next day with the power coming back on about 10:00 am. We finally decided to head back to civilization where we could ensure the Jell-O would stay cold.

This week will bring only one interaction with the medical community. They are putting in my PICC line (Peripherally Inserted Central Catheter) on Thursday. This involves putting an IV in my arm at about the elbow and running it up and across the shoulder until it reaches the vein draining the head. This will allow the introduction of the chemo drugs into a larger vein where it will dilute faster. I understand that this reduces the chances of damaging the veins and surrounding tissue in the arm. Sounds like a good idea to me. I'll just have to hold off on my Tour d' France training program. This training program starts with tasting as many French wines as I can find. You can't be racing around France without knowing your first growths.

Next chemotherapy starts next Monday. They will be treating me once every four weeks with cisplatin (the same old drug I had during radiation) and 5-FU. The cisplatin is given in a single session (takes about five hours). You get to go home with the 5-FU strapped to your arm and dripping slowly into your vein. This takes five days. They say, "it's not called 5-FU for nothing." I'm sure I'll figure that out none too soon.

It's so quiet around here. I need my kids. Love, Mike

Chapter 48

I've Been Saved Before

"Save Carter"
- PRick Bacher (the "P" is silent)

Once upon a time, in a far away land, there was a boy named Mike. Just like all nerds, he had some issues in high school. Actually, the high school was fine; it was the other students in the school that caused his struggles. These struggles varied from always being the last one picked in gym to the normal teasing from Jock to Nerd. The apex of the struggles manifested itself in the most dreaded of all school activities (with the exception of school dances) - Dodgeball. Everyone knows the drill – the jocks pummel the nerds showing their supreme mastery of all things important to getting the chicks. This was more than your average Dodgeball - this was worse than normal. There were the normal share of Jocks in school: The Hill Twins (Jim and Tim), PRick Bacher (The P is silent), and the future famous Rich Dudsin. Rich became a pitcher for the Chicago White Sox with a 98 mph fastball and some serious attitude. "Famous" is relative. He's likely the most "famous" person from Anderson High School but "famous?" A signed baseball with his name on it is worth $12.95 plus the cost of the ink - and you have to pay for shipping and handling.

For some reason, Jocks hate Nerds. Dodgeball provided the perfect forum for working out their issues. The rules were simple enough for even the Jockiest to remember. Selection of weapons (the dodgeballs) was crucial. One little-known rule that was never written down but certainly observed in practice: only the jocks can catch and throw the balls. The standard issue ball assortment ranged from beach-ball-sized ball with maximum speed about 5 mph down to a grapefruit-sized projectile capable of speeds approaching 100 mph in the hands of barbarians like Jim, Tim, Rich and PRick (the P is silent).

The dodgeball rules were probably not that different from what you know. When you get hit – you are out. If you catch someone's throw – they are out. The game was played on the basketball court and started with no one allowed to cross the half-court line. The early game was not that bad and after a few dodgeball sessions, the nerd's strategy cleverly shifts from "try to catch and throw" to "get hit early" to avoid the end-game. The challenge for the nerds was to get hit quickly without making it look like they were trying to get out early. If they got caught, the gym teacher would yell out, "Carter! You're in for good!" Oh how that would touch the heart of the callous jock. The other chant heard frequently on those rainy dodgeball days was, "Save Carter!" How kind of them to save a nerd for the slaughter at the end of the game. Mike used to pray for sunshine so he could stay inside and play chess with a teacher. The Jocks seemed to pray for rain. Mike's only solace - the "P" is silent.

Half way through the game, the future Nobel-Peace-Prize-winning gym teacher would yell out "Foul Line" allowing the assailants to cross half court and go all the way to the foul line in their search for the perfect game. A few minutes later one would hear the former-junior-high-regional-wrestling-champion-genius turned "teacher" shout - "Baseline!" allowing all players full access to the entire court and most importantly, point blank range for the nerd kill. This is where the "Save Carter" strategy was most effective as they would encircle the remaining fetal nerd body, each with a ball and countdown "3, 2, 1…"

Those bastards work for Mike now… "3, 2, 1… work!"

A few years after high school, we went to Coney Island swimming pool one summer day. Coney Island is (or was) the site for the world's largest recirculation swimming pool. The pool had multiple diving boards including a three-meter platform. There was also a concrete island in the middle of the pool. I ran into PRick (the P is silent) Bacher out near the island. He says, "Get Carter" and proceeds to dunk me and hold me under for what seemed like a minute. In hindsight, it wasn't much longer than 50 seconds. Man, do I wish he worked for me now…

It confirmed one thing: the "P" is still silent.

Chapter 49

Time Flies When You're being Tortured

"Never, never, never give up."
- Sir Winston Churchill

August 10, 2003

This is my 18*th* weekly update. Hard to believe it's been that long since this all started. Time flies when you're being tortured. I've chosen a new font this week in a feeble attempt to remove the strange signs replacing my apostrophes (we're going to try Helvetica). All you PC users out there – let me know if this helps. It must be a pain to read these with the font screwed up. Sorry – my first complaint didn't come until this last week (Thanks Ed W.).

First, I'd like to announce my official withdrawal as candidate for Governor of California. The 65 validated signatures and $3,500 were not the issue. Neither was Arnold or Gallagher or Father Guido Sarduchi, or Larry Flint, or the 100 year-old woman, or the porn star. I just didn't think I could beat Gary Coleman. Yeah, I'm taller and clearly could carry the physicist vote but the short, former child actor crowd is a tough lobby to go up against. All those munchkins! I might decide to run a write-in campaign. With more than 150 people on the ballot and a "Recall Arnold" campaign already started, I think all bets are off. A baseball commissioner – get real – it's just a game! I need a slogan. How about an environmental, save the redwoods theme with slogan "read my lips, no new axes?"

This week saw another access port installed in my body. This time it's a PICC line. The installation is pretty straightforward (except in my case). I felt like an Egyptian King: lying on the procedure bed – nurse working my right arm – Laura fanning me with moistened branches as I tried to keep from fainting. They insert the catheter into your arm and run it up your vein, into the chest where your veins converge and head for the heart. After the procedure, they sent me down to radiology to double check the installation. On the way through the crowded lobby of the *hospital, I was stopped by a nurse who asked me if I was all right. I did not look good. I think she wanted the short version of the story. Oh well, I swear I could feel the line in my shoulder and chest (you are not supposed to feel anything).*

In radiology, they put a lead shield on me (yeah – who needs that?) and took a radiograph – and guess what – It's in two inches too far. Looking at the diagram – two inches sounds like "in the heart" to me. They pulled it out a bit (I got fanned some more) and off we went.

The next day we realized that my jugular veins on the right side have been removed. I wonder if they knew that when they chose the right arm? We'll have to ask on Monday.

Tomorrow (Monday) the counter-attack begins. I start my second round of Chemotherapy. The PICC line should make this easier. I get the same old drug Cisplatin on Monday (one dose every four weeks) and I get to go home with the 5-FU pump strapped to my arm for five days. Rumor is that they warn you: if the 5-FU spills – DO NOT TOUCH IT! – It's poison! It's ok to drip it into the vein just above the heart but don't touch it? It works for me...

I'm optimistic that the chemotherapy will not be quite as bad this week. I now realize that much of the nausea was from the phlegm and the phlegm was "caused" by the radiation to the throat. I've gotten Fred to go on vacation and Ethel's visits are manageable. There is some reason for optimism here but we'll see come Wednesday or Thursday if the two chemotherapy drugs (Ricky and Lucy) will draw Fred and Ethel back to the apartment. This makes little sense... I guess I've got some splainin to do.

Not much else to update on this week. Kids are still gone and Laura and I are tired of interacting with only each other. We're really gonna suffer from the empty nest syndrome when David goes off to college. We have seven years to work a strategy – we'd better start this next week.

Eating is going well. I still have the feeding tube and use it every day. Still having trouble gaining weight. At least I'm stable –

scrawny but stable. I haven't been worried about the diet. It consists primarily of eggs, butter, salmon, salt, sugar, filet, and King crab legs double dipped in melted butter. I'll worry about the cholesterol when the kids are away at college. This week saw me venture out to the Thai, Chinese and Italian restaurants of the tri-valley. I'm slow but I can eat!

Until next week, I miss you all! It's so quiet around here – I hope Arnold comes by.

Love, Mike

Chapter 50

Train Wreck

"To boldly go where no man has gone before."
 - Captain James Tiberius Kirk

Laura and I first met when we were undergraduates at Indiana University in Bloomington, Indiana. I had gone to Indiana as a music major in the fall of 1976. The story about my change of major at the end of my freshman year (to physics) can be read (or skipped) elsewhere in this book. Laura's freshman year as a math major began in the fall a year later. Her first year was Mike-free, but in the fall of 1978 a mutual friend and calculus mate, Dave Dortch, had "introduced" us at a distance. Dave was in my calculus class and he lived on the floor below Laura in her double-tower, eleven-story dormitory. Laura and I knew of each other through Dave and "studied together" through Dave without actually meeting. Dave had also talked me into working at the cafeteria in Briscoe Hall. Laura and I finally met one morning as I carried a pan of scrambled eggs out to the serving line. She was making toast for the masses. It was hardly a "love at first sight" moment. Both of us were proudly wearing our hairnets and red and white-checkered cafeteria uniforms. What's not to love? On the other hand – maybe eggs and toast go together.

Our relationship got off to a bit of a rough start when I failed to show at her birthday party in late October. It wasn't like we had a relationship. I had a girlfriend in Cincinnati and every time I had seen Laura, she was wearing the same outfit: the cafeteria uniform. A couple months later, I was invited to a Christmas party that she and her friends were having just before we all left for Christmas break. I decided to go and bring my girlfriend from Cincinnati.

The party was memorable for two reasons: homemade fudge, and a telltale comment from my girlfriend in the stairwell after the party. In one of the classic tipping points in life, Laura had drawn my name for the gift exchange and had given me a Steve Martin comedy album and plate of her mother's homemade fudge. Now, unbeknownst to me, Laura's Mom doesn't make fudge the way our family makes fudge. We make the marshmallow cream kind that any idiot can make. I find out later that Laura's Mom is a phenomenal, old-fashioned cook and makes fudge the old-fashioned way – by hand – from scratch. It's way different from our fudge and, so I hear, it tastes very, very good.

There is one significant problem: I like the marshmallow cream kind. I gave the precious plate of hand-crafted fudge to my girlfriend (while we were at the party). My children owe their existence to my future wife who could see beyond these early party fouls. I had not really noticed much of the interpersonal dynamic at the party but as my girlfriend and I were walking down the stairwell from the 11th floor of my future wife's dormitory, I asked her how she liked my friends. Her response was the first sign that I needed a train derailment. "Laura really likes you."

"Does she?" I replied. I kind of like her too… that checkered uniform… and hairnet… (I didn't say any of that out loud but I think I thought it.)

"How can you tell?" I asked, like a guy paying close attention to the world around him.

"I can just tell," she replied. (I guess girls can "just tell.")

Christmas break didn't clear anything up at all. My girlfriend and I were revving the train – talking of marriage and transfer to the University of Cincinnati. I returned to Indiana in January and found myself spending time with Laura – now occasionally without the hairnet. She seemed unattainable. Our excuses to spend time together were studying and watching MASH. Just after one of the episodes (probably where Major Frank Burns and Margaret "Hot Lips" Houlihan kissed) I decided to give Laura that first kiss (on the cheek). Anything else would have been a move way too far forward. Little did I know this was Laura's first kiss. Clearly, others had been scared off long before this point. Boy did I ever understand that. For some reason that I still can't write down - she was scary. She didn't scream (or really respond much at all) but I could tell there was a train wreck coming and increasingly I wanted it.

Enter stage right: the Valentine's Day Massacre. My girlfriend came to Bloomington for the Valentine's Day weekend and it was increasingly clear to both of us (or at least me) that we were through. She and I parted ways that weekend – broken up. She received some lovely parting gifts – flowers, candy and a Valentine's card. But they were just that – parting gifts. It was over. Now I could turn my attention to Laura. The first opportunity to have a positive impact was blown. If I would have chosen a card, or flowers, or a box of candy (or some marshmallow cream fudge) to give her on Valentine's Day, I would have been golden. But living in fear of failure (or fear of success) I went with the most memorable of all Valentine-day gifts – nothing. My kids owe Laura another debt of gratitude for her tolerance of complete romantic incompetence. This was the first of many consecutive Valentine's Day fiascos. I'm just cursed around mid-February. To this day, every February I seek out conferences, meetings, and contagious diseases to attempt to avoid the inevitable. Luckily for me, Laura loves me for something else. Something we have yet to identify. I should adopt a "don't ask, don't tell" policy.

Our first real date was a sign of wonderful things to come. We walked to dinner and a movie at the theater south of the university. It had rained earlier in the day. Laura seized this opportunity to jump into a puddle, splashing her future groom with muddy rainwater (this would later become one of our kids' favorite bedtime stories). We then enjoyed dinner in the fine restaurant (Mr. Steak) at the corner of Third Street and the Bypass, Laura looking out the window counting the busses that stopped at the bus stop just outside. The movie was quite memorable – the first Star Trek movie. It started with the 20-minute-long sequences surveying the outside of the USS Enterprise. That was even a bit much for the Star Trek lover in me. Laura has absolutely no love for Captain James T. Kirk and the beloved crew of the USS Enterprise (NCC-1701). She probably wishes they all wore red shirts.

Chapter 51

Hiccups

"If you're [still] going through hell, keep going."
 - Sir Winston Churchill

August 17, 2003

This is my 19th weekly update. Is anyone getting tired of these yet (other than me)? I hope they are as much fun to read as they are to write. Especially this week. Hey, at least we had power all week. This was an interesting week where we ran out of characters to name the side effects. Maybe we should have chosen Petticoat Junction instead of I Love Lucy. Billy Jo, Betty Jo, and Bobby Jo could have split the Phlegm and chronic dry mouth. Uncle Jo could have been the symbol of loss of sex drive. Steve (yeah – Oneofthe Jo's husband) could have been my weight loss symbol. Still looking for a symbol for the hiccups – maybe the damn dog. (This will become important later in the week.)

The week started like all great weeks in California, beautiful sunny weather, and a coastal breeze cooling the valley every night. The kids are off at Camp in Minnesota fending off the Minnesota state bird swarms and having the times of their young lives. Add in a little visit to the doctor who lifts our spirits by saying our prognosis is "excellent." (He comes to this conclusion by "listening to my lungs" and submitting the paperwork for scheduling an MRI.) Hey, he must be very good (or we must be suckers for taking in any bits of good news in our desperate situation). He does point out that my red blood cell count is low and we'll be starting a reddie upper tomorrow ($1,800 drug for four injections) – but I'm worth it.

The chemotherapy process is like eating an old piece of cake. The cisplatin goes in the PICC line like a fine 10-40W at the Oil Changers. No filters to change just add some fluids to control the nausea. Our confidence is high, we've done cisplatin before and they have lowered the dose. They add a continuous arm pump of *the 5-FU and send us home. Laura drives and I don't stress – life is good.*

We spent most of the week resting (lots of sleeping and eating). Not bad for a chemo week. The kids returned home on Thursday night from their family environmental camp north of Lake Superior and we were all back together again. Our kids have been absolutely wonderful to Laura and me as we work through this year of road bumps. We're gonna do something great as a family when this gets settled down just a bit. Hawaii, a cruise, a week at the library – something we can all enjoy.

On Friday, we took out the 5-FU – (no sign of any additional side effects), pulled out the PICC line to mentally increase my mobility in my right arm, and listened to the advise of the chemotherapy nurses. "Yeah – you can back off on the anti-nausea drugs, you're over the hump." Now – what were we thinking????

Friday night, the hiccups "Little Ricky" (the only character left in I Love Lucy) reared his ugly head and would not shut up. A friend in Washington, DC had warned me that uncontrolled hiccups could be a problem. A PROBLEM! Britney Spears' wardrobe is a problem. Sparing the details about how to break the hiccups other than vomiting (spared because I know no other way). I'll just summarize by saying – it was a really bad weekend. Little Ricky returned twice on Saturday and is not welcome in this house again. I ended up with a diaphragm so sore I could barely sit up. Eating was relegated to the bare minimum and I was not the best of patients. Finally, as Monday morning rolls around, I appear to be getting back on top of it (with the anti-nausea meds back in the plan). We'll wean off them a little more slowly next time.

We missed a family wedding on Mackinac Island this weekend that would have been a lot of fun. It's just a short ferry ride from St. Ignace Michigan just over the Mackinaw Bridge. It's real easy to get to (once you are there). My cousin Susan, one of the funnest persons in the world, surely missed my dancing prowess. I dance like a 130-pound nerd from the 70s (and now I almost look like one again).

Laura has been a real trooper – I could NOT survive this without her – of this I am absolutely sure. There are times when I feel I can't go on. You want to tell the docs "enough is enough – I can't do this." She's there to give me the gentle encouragement I need to suck it up and plow ahead. Is she a little too happy about Uncle Jo? – Not yet but he'll be asleep on the front porch in a few months. Until next week, may Little Ricky bless someone else's house?

Love, Mike

Chapter 52

Engaged

"Will you marry me?"
- Every Groom but me

I am not well known for my romance. This is a debatable fact but so is most everything. I blame my romantic tendencies on my wife. Her definition of romance and mine must be different. Our "proposal" is one example.

We were in the "just dating" phase of our relationship in college and she had decided to get her wisdom teeth pulled. Being the loyal, dedicated, and committed boyfriend that I was, I offered to take her and sit in the waiting room during the surgery and of course, drive her home safely after the procedure. After an hour or so of waiting patiently in the reception area and reading every National Geographic I could find, the door opened and the nurse came out to get someone to go back to the recovery room and sit with Laura as the drugs wore off.

There were three or four of us in the waiting room so, there are witnesses. The nurse asked, "Is Laura Helmond's fiancé here?" I glanced around and noticed that no one else was standing up. I quickly realized – that must be me. I guess we're engaged. Who says drugs aren't a good thing?

The rest is history. We were married on my 23rd birthday in May of 1981. It was a very memorable ceremony. Laura's Uncle Bob performed the ceremony at the Methodist church in Plainfield Indiana. After the vows, ring exchange, and kiss, Uncle Bob introduced us to our families and friends as "Mr. and Mrs. Michael Roberts." Laura's family catered the reception at her Mom and Dad's house and, as always, the food was simple and spectacular. Laura's mother, Emma Jean, made all the food. Aunt Ruth made the wedding and groom's cakes. The groom's cake was the family specialty: chocolate cake with homemade caramel icing.

Two days later we loaded up the yellow, 1974 Chevy Beauville Sportvan and moved to California. We were on our own: No debt - no money – no plants – no furniture – no pets. All we needed was that lamp. Navin R. Johnson ("The Jerk") would have been proud.

Chapter 53

Mrs. McGillicuddy

"We have drugs for that."
- Best Nurse Ever!

August 24, 2003

Update #20. This was an interesting week. I must admit, I was not prepared for this phase of chemotherapy to be so darn difficult (especially week two of the monthly cycle). By the way, I'd like to thank everyone who sent in obscure characters from the I Love Lucy Show – now I can develop more side effects – I was almost out of nicknames.

This week it was – Mrs. McGillicuddy (better known as hypochondria). Now don't get me wrong, obsession with symptoms can be a good thing. Right? Well, this week I went through multiple symptoms and for each, identified the likely cause:

- sore throat – recurrent throat cancer

- constipation – colon cancer

- shortness of breath – lung cancer

- lack of skin color – liver cancer

- mouth sores – tongue cancer

- runny nose – nasal cancer

- neuropathy – some kind of nerve cancer – probably brain

- sore hip – bone cancer

- dehydration – water cancer – (cancer of the hydrogenous tissues)

Guess what the advice nurse says, if you can get them to pick up the phone... "Sorry, you must have the wrong number." (Actually – "drink more water!" and "we have drugs for that.")

I think you get the idea. The symptoms are real. Their cause is – who knows? My guess is – I don't know – the poison they dump in my veins? The fact is that waiting to get SOME data on whether this treatment regimen is working or not can be a grueling psychological tour de force. It's much more difficult to handle than I thought it would be.

In the mean time, I am actually feeling better this weekend – most of the above-mentioned cancers are on holiday along with the French grape pickers. Let's hope only the grape harvest comes in early.

I'm preparing arguments for the doctor about the next chemotherapy round. I need either less poison or more of those "drugs for that" that they talk about. First step was to get a year's supply of hiccup-stopper medicine. Hey – it says it stops the hiccups (which I have not had since last weekend) and causes a very long list of other side effects. But when you have the hiccups, you would trade your ____(fill in the blank) to get rid of them!

It's hard to believe, but doctors use Body Surface Area to calculate your chemotherapy dose. They even give it an acronym (BSA). That's why I've decided to soak myself in a cold bath before my next appointment. The coefficient of thermal expansion of human skin is currently being measured (I've dumped ice in the hot tub) and I'm going to take the data. I'm just not going to take this high dose crap anymore! (Unless Laura or the doctors say I have to.)

I found a news article on the web this weekend: "Biologists have found a class of chemicals that they hope will make people live longer by activating an ancient survival reflex. One of the chemicals, a natural substance known as resveratrol, is found in red wines, particularly those made in cooler climates like that of New York."

If this doesn't read like NIH Pork from Senator Clinton's district, then what does? Just in case, I'm buying wines from the far northern reaches of the Napa Valley.

Not much else to add this week. Kids start school this coming Wednesday. Big steps for both – Sarah is starting 9th grade and David is starting middle school. The kids are ready. There is a three day weekend coming up – I wonder if I'll notice. Every day is a three-day weekend for me these days.

Until next week – We may rest assured that water cancer is not in my future!

Love, Mike

Chapter 54

2:07:43

"Dad! You Cheat!"
- Sarah and David Carter

In 2002, my mother and I spent the weekend in New York City. It was one of those wonderful experiences in life – just me and Mom. We stayed at the chic W Hotel just off Times Square. We had a great dinner at the Brazilian steakhouse on 57th street in Midtown Manhattan. We saw the Broadway show Chicago, before the movie came out. If was a beautiful fall weekend: one that neither of us will ever forget. We watched the NFL Live broadcast with Neon Deion Sanders in an outdoor studio at the edge of Central Park. He looks even better in person than on TV. We also had the opportunity to watch the New York City Marathon. I had never had an interest in watching Kenyans run circles around the Americans, but being there in person I noticed that marathon runners don't run in circles and they are very, very impressive athletes. It's hard to believe they run faster at mile 24 than I can in a 100-yard dash.

Fast forward a year and I'm now sitting in my California home, trying to recover and watching the New York City Marathon "live" on TV. I called the kids down and told them that Grandma and I had been there last year and it was sort of fun to watch. I challenged them to estimate the finish time: closest time wins! I took the first guess – 2:07:43.

The kids immediately boxed me in. Dave took 2:07:44. Sarah took 2:07:42. As the race came close to its finish, they cheered for the leader: over or under 2:07:43 and one of them would win (and they would both be happy – anything to beat Dad!). The first Kenyan crossed the line: time = 2:07:43. Dad nailed it! Brilliant guess! The thrill of Victory! The kids were stunned. I did my favorite victory dance in the living room. Life was good.

(The race was being broadcast on a three-hour tape delay in California – I had looked up the winning time on the Internet.)

Life was good!

To be clear: I had a policy with my kids – It is ok to lie to me IF you are 100% certain you are going to get caught.

As a corollary to this story, every Christmas we travel to the Midwest to visit my family in Cincinnati and Laura's family in Plainfield, Indiana. We have only missed this annual trip twice: once in 1981 when, as newlyweds, we had no money; and once in 1989 when Laura was pregnant with Sarah and the doctors advised us that Christmas was too close to the due date to travel across the country.

Every year we drive back and forth between our parents' homes. It's about a two hour and nineteen minute drive. One of the games we play is to guess the arrival time at Granny's house in Plainfield. It is not unusual to find me driving five miles per hour for the last mile or two just to do everything I can to win!

Winning is fun but, with my kids, it's always more fun to get caught cheating.

Chapter 55

Forgive me Father

"There's a big difference between "20 years of experience" and "An experience that lasted 20 years"."
- B. J. McKinley

September 1, 2003

Update #21. Finally, September has arrived. I decided to take a holiday and send this update out on Tuesday morning instead of the normal Monday distribution. This has been a good week. I don't think I've felt this well since April. Then again, I don't remember what I felt like before the treatments began. As I recall, I felt OK but the good memories fade with the bad.

Looking back at last week's note, I can't believe how much progress I've made in a week. No mythical diseases, no I Love Lucy characters (occasional visit from Ethel but... that's a long-term problem). What a difference a week makes.

Oh, before I forget... Forgive me father, for I have sinned. Sinned, maybe but I also have scored an MRI appointment. Although not mentioned explicitly in the 10 commandments, I assume lying to the radiology department is a sin. It turns out they had somehow lost the request from my doctor to get me scanned and had no time to get me in until after the turn of the next millennium. I gave them this big song and dance about how the doctor needed the results of the scan before my next chemotherapy on the 8th of September. They fell for it like a climber when his protection comes loose. So – I'm in on the 5th. Should be a fun hour in the tube. Thinking back to the previous MRI, I think drugs are in order before this one. All that caving when I was young should help me through this one (but drugs are good too).

Other big news in California – I got out with Randy Bell (a friend from DC) and played nine holes of golf on Sunday. I started out the first hole with a birdie. If that's not big news, I don't know what is. I should take advantage of the free time and work on my golf game.

The kids have their first three days of school behind them. In fine family form, David missed day two (he was being visited by Ricky). Luckily, day two of sixth grade is not a big deal to miss. He was back to full speed by the afternoon on Thursday so we went and signed him up for guitar lessons. That is just what we need around the house – more noise.

I'll keep this one short for a change. Hope all is well around the country.

Love, Mike

Chapter 56

Dear John

*"The difference between a good physicist and a bad physicist is –
A bad physicist can't tell what's not important."*
- B. J. McKinley

Sometimes, we make mistakes. Sometimes, they are big mistakes. Sometimes they are just mistakes in judgment. Sometimes these mistakes go unnoticed – even by us – sometimes not. They often come back to bite us… sometimes right away, sometimes not. Sometimes, what seems like a mistake might not be. Sometimes, what seems like it is not a mistake might indeed be one. It's complicated. Immune from these "mistakes," I am not.

As I have mentioned before, I was honored to work in the Transition Planning Office for the standup of the Department of Homeland Security in the fall of 2002. I sat in a cubicle overlooking the National Mall in a nondescript office building just one block from the White House. Across the aisle from my cube was a fellow scientist, Dr. John Vitko. John was from Sandia National Laboratory's Livermore campus. We had met before we were sent to Washington but I didn't know John very well. We were just competing scientists at competing National Laboratories.

John was in charge of the Biosecurity R&D plan and I was in charge of the Radiological & Nuclear Security R&D plan. Between the two of us we "owned" the biggest share of the R&D program in DHS. We quickly became colleagues and friends. John was a driven but polite scientist with never a cruel word to say about anyone. John had a sense of class about him that I was missing. Maybe something to learn someday, but I was too busy to focus on such less important attributes. My style was much less formal – more working-class collegial.

I developed a habit, something men occasionally do, of giving John the finger whenever I saw him. It was given as a friendly gesture – a "sign of affection." John would smile and return the gesture with a kind word or two. "Good morning, Carter" or "I love you too" would not be uncommon. It became habit on both sides of the aisle: me and my crude gesture (a sign of affection), he and his kind words. They could coexist in harmony: for a while.

While back in California undergoing cancer treatment John and his wife Kitty, came to visit. Again I was found in my pajamas, hiding my feeding tube, anxious to get caught up on the events in the new Department of Homeland Security. Laura did not know John or Kitty but had heard many (but not all) stories about John and our adventures in Government. John proceeded to recount the story he told his two teenage daughters during the 2002 Christmas break.

John, now telling this story to Laura (with Kitty laughing) says, "There is a guy at work that, every time he sees me, gives me the finger." John's daughters apparently think this is the funniest thing they have ever heard. Their father has apparently never cussed or given the famous gesture to anyone – not even while driving on the freeways in California. I'm wondering if there is something wrong with John. (Laura is wondering if there is something wrong with me).

John proceeds to tell us that he is an Elder in the Russian Orthodox Church and, upon his retirement from government service, he plans to study to become a priest. This explains John and his ways of interacting with others. He works under a different set of rules – guided by a higher power. He also understands me. John knows what's important.

Chapter 57

Asti Spumante?

"Everyone has his day and some days last longer than others."
- Sir Winston Churchill

September 7, 2003

Update #22. OK – first things first. We have received some good news. Now before we break into song, the first read of the MRI from the radiologist (probably the same one that botched the read in May) was very positive. I had called my surgeon (Dr. Eye Contact, M.D.) and asked him to review it ASAP. He called this morning at 8:00am – again showing that he speaks very well if eye contact is not required. They both agree – the tumor in the parapharyngeal space is gone and there is no sign of cancer anywhere in the head and neck region. It doesn't get any better than that.

Second things second – chemotherapy continues. After receiving news last week that my blood count was too low to proceed, they scheduled me for a 7:00am blood draw on Monday morning with the idea that my count would improve enough to begin round two. Fortunately (I guess), I was deemed fit to go and they began the 7-hour ordeal at 8:30 this morning. The first attempts to get the PICC line in resulted only in a significant blood letting from the right arm. I asked for the leeches to be added too, but the nurse didn't think that was very funny. As our experience has shown it was time for two changes – move to the left arm and get a new nurse. Nurse two was successful; the radiograph showed the PICC in the right place and – dripping of the poison began by 11:00 am.

The MRI (last Friday) was significantly easier than the previous scan from hell. I still had issues with their "don't swallow for the next twelve minutes" commands. I just can't keep the throat from trying to swallow even though there is nothing to swallow. It's only a partially voluntary action and I wasn't in complete command. We made it with only a small amount of image blurring. One hundred minutes in the tube is just about enough. I found the rarest item in the hospital – a compassionate Radiation Technician. I wore my President of the United State golf shirt and I think she was confused about who I was and how important I might be. She actually seemed to care as she rolled me in the tube with final instructions "do not move for the next one hundred minutes." Hey at least she said it in a nice tone of voice.

My Oncologist (a champion of minimizing the severity of side effects that he has never experienced) assures me that after October's chemotherapy, they will leave me alone... Finally, I have something to look forward to in the world of chemotherapy.

Now the challenge is to keep focused on completing this chemotherapy while the MRI's show no sign of cancer. I hope I can do it. Without Laura and my family and friends, I have no shot.

Almost time to break out the good stuff (not the Asti Spumante). These next two weeks will be tough but we're plowing ahead. Thanks Laura and Ellen.

Love, Mike

Chapter 58

A Nearly Null Set

"You learn more from failure than success."
- Steve Patterson

You may wonder why I don't speak much about our family pets. There is a reason. We are mostly pet-free in the Carter household with a few important exceptions. To start, I grew up with a family dog, Penny. Penny had her challenges but we really loved her. She did the dog thing in a time when dogs were free to chase cars, bark at mailmen, chase kids on bikes, fetch the paper (which she never did), and just roam around doing their thing. Laura, on the other hand, must have come from a family of "being chased." Many years ago, Laura made me choose between her and pets. In hindsight, I guess I chose wisely. Although, a dog can be quite comforting when you are not feeling well.

There are two important exceptions to our family's "no pet" rule. Many years ago, during one of my Monday through Thursday trips to Washington DC, Laura and the kids bought a goldfish bowl, two goldfish, fish food and whatever else goldfish need. Being contained in the fishbowl ensured that the goldfish would not chase cars, mailmen, or kids on bikes without the constraints of the pet leash. Leash laws in California are very strict. In the time it took me to travel and return home, the family bought the fish, both fish died and they threw everything away. I never saw the fish, the bowl, the food, or the crying kids. They recovered but have yet to enjoy the companionship a goldfish or dog could have provided. Inspiring, you say? It gets better.

The kids would often ask me (not Laura) – "Can we get a dog? " I always said we'd have to trade in Mom (maybe not in exactly those words). Somehow, inspired by a dose of boldness, while I was on a trip to DC in very early April of 1997, David (at age five) stepped forward. I called one night from the hotel and David proceeded to inform me that he and Sarah had talked Mom into getting a dog. They had the dog home and it was going great. It was a puppy, brown, fun, etc… all the things you expect a five year old to say about the new family pet. I was on the other end of the phone in complete shock. Somewhere between "Wow – I love dogs" and "Do I really have to give up Laura now?" I just don't have a clue what to say. I'm asking questions and he has answers to everything… and then he blurts out… "April Fools!"

Got me… Got me good… Bested by a five-year-old... No dog.

We get to keep Laura… Life is good.

Chapter 59

Clear MRI

"I've had worse."
- Black Knight

"You Liar."
- King Arthur, Monty Python and the Holy Grail

September 15, 2003

Update #23. This has been a very quiet week after receiving the great news about the clear MRI. The chemotherapy proceeded as scheduled with the dominant side effect being extreme fatigue. Sleeping eighteen hours a day does make the time go faster. My second chemotherapy drug (the dreaded 5-FU) strapped to my arm for a slow week of infusion, ran out a little fast so I got the PICC line pulled out a day early. Nice to have full arm movement back and be free to shower.

Little Ricky (the hiccups) returned right on schedule Friday evening. This time, I was prepared with relaxed breathing and drugs! Relaxed breathing is something like Lamaze. It makes you feel better, helps you relax but isn't going to stop that little Ricky from coming in the end. This time, the drugs seemed to help and Ricky's two-day visit wasn't nearly as bad as last month. Diaphragm a little sore and afraid to breathe and swallow, but I'm still a functioning person.

Not much going on on the home front. Laura and kids still standing right there by me every step of the way. If I were her, I'd be really tired of rubbing my neck but somehow, in her ongoing competition with Mother Theresa, she never complains. Meals typically consist of three or four separate entrees (when you consider what David and I eat - "entrees.") We just push through it and do our best.

I keep looking at the light at the end of the tunnel and thinking I should describe "life out there" before I really see it. Kind of like making new years' predictions and resolutions but get it down on paper. I know much will be the same (work deadlines, school studies and taxi service) but much will change. I have a renewed sense of appreciation for my family and friends and hopefully the finer things in life (there goes my wine bill). We just can't waste an evening with Two-Buck Chuck. The one thing that never changes is the rate time carries us along. I've got to remember that somehow. (I'll probably get 30 physicist friends reminding me of the theory of relativity and that I'm not exactly correct, but we'll leave that for the Professor and Mary Ann on the next episode of "Sit-Com Cancer"). They will never get off that Island.

Not much on the medical front ahead this week. No doctors, just recover from the 5-FU. Expect a week of "small side effects" – fatigue, sore mouth, nausea, diarrhea, you know, easy stuff. If my last chemotherapy in October is only this bad – I can take it. (I can take it if it's worse too but – I DON'T WANT TO!)

The doctor signed paperwork for me to start back to work part time on the 22nd. I'm looking forward to my two hours per day for the first two weeks. We'll see how that goes. At two hours a day it's just like taking the full eight hours off and just working a bit of overtime. I never got anything done until those last two hours anyhow. Sounds like a new alternate work plan to me.

Until next week, keep the emails coming; I really enjoy hearing from everyone even if I don't respond to every reply. You all give me strength to carry on. We're going to make it and see what life is like outside this tunnel! It's going to be better than ever!

Love, Mike

Chapter 60

Cactus Carter

"It was something I ate or something I drank."
- Mike Carter

Back in the days of nuclear testing, I spent a lot of time at the Nevada Test Site (NTS). The Laboratory operated an airplane ("AMI") flying back and forth from the Livermore airport to the Desert Rock airport at Mercury Nevada every day. It was not unusual to fly up to NTS every Monday morning and back to Livermore on Friday afternoon. We spent many hours at NTS with very little to do other than to work and explore the test site. There are many memorable stories but if you ask my friends from that era, nearly everyone can tell the story about how I got my nickname – "Cactus Carter."

While at the site, we were issued government cars but were forbidden from leaving the site unless you had official business in Las Vegas. In the event of such business, you were issued a car pass (pink card) and could "get out of jail free." This imprisonment was not so bad for the first few months but after a while, you really felt trapped. During the CONTACT shot preparations, the crafts went on strike. This included the cafeteria workers, so the food selection was limited to what you could buy out of the vending machines (chili, frozen burritos, popcorn). This was extremely limiting – so, we made up a story about a meeting in Vegas and scored some pink cards one evening. Off we went – 4-5 cars full of guys to Cactus Springs!

Cactus Springs was/is just a wide spot in the road a few miles from Indian Springs with nothing more than a bar and a sign along the road. We were, of course, careful to park our government cars around the back side of the bar (away from the road) to avoid the obvious "6 government cars parked in front of the bar" syndrome. We were just hoping for pizza and a few beers. Instead – It was Schnapps night - $1 a shot. The guys got me started playing pool for shots of Schnapps. A few simple lessons were learned that night: You can't beat Jack Robson and Tom Schaffer at their own game and after the first dozen shots of schnapps, they all taste like peach! (Oh – and be careful with Johanna Swan – she may call your bluff).

The next day was interesting. We were installing and doing the final check of some high-tech detectors on the shot and I think the guys needed me (it was my responsibility). I was not in the best shape. We were working on the 7th and 8th floors of the tower (a modular, ten story metal "building" constructed around the canister). There were two ways to get up and down the tower. One was a tight spiral staircase in the corner of the tower, the other was a freight/passenger elevator attached to the outside of the building. The only "restrooms" were porta-potties across the gravel parking lot from the tower. Well, needless to say, it takes a long time to get from level 8 to the porta-potties to throw-up. There is one other option – use your hardhat. That's how I got the nickname "Cactus Carter."

Later that day, with a good week's work behind me, I headed for Mercury to catch AMI back to Livermore. I still was not at the top of my game and that was going to hurt me. AMI took off from Desert Rock airstrip and flew low and slow over the hot thermals of the Nevada Desert, over the Sierras at about 18,000 ft and then down into Livermore. The flight was low and slow across the screaming hot foothills into a 40 mph wind. Nice smooth sailing it was not!

I was sitting right next to a brand new guy in my world (rare – we all knew everyone). Denny Chakedis was the new mechanical technician supervisor (all my techs worked for him). Denny was a veteran of the test site but he had worked programs I was not associated with. Denny was a caring, hard-ass Greek (if you know the type). If you're friends with Denny – you're friends with Denny. If not – he was a real hard-ass. Well, we were about 200 feet off the end of the tarmac, enjoying the thermals upon assent over the Nevada desert and I didn't have my hardhat. Denny and I were not friends yet. But Denny's techs (specifically the previously mentioned Jack and Tom) had several hobbies. One hobby apparently was to cut small holes in the bottom of the barf bags on AMI. Funny! Woo! So, as my barf bag dripped onto my brand-new Gortex jacket, Denny asks me if I'm ok. My response, "it was either something I ate or something I drank." I should have said, "It was Jack and Tom."

Denny and I became good friends. Denny passed away from a heart attack before retiring. He worked hard every day of his life. Denny also worked with the Lab's education program bringing science and technology education to Native American children across the southwest. Denny continues to be a role model for me. I see his smiling face in a picture on the wall of the conference room at the Livermore office building in Washington, DC. Also smiling is the kid, blowing on a straw, inflating a ziplock bag and lifting a lead brick. We all miss you Denny!

Jack and Tom were masters of the practical joke. When back at Livermore working at my office I had struggled with my desk chair. Every day I would come to work and the pneumatic cylinder used to adjust the height of the chair needed to be raised. I thought the cylinder just had a small leak - hardly worth complaining about. Every day for about six months I would come to work, raise my chair back up to its working height and get started. One day I made the mistake of coming in to work about an hour early and I discovered the problem. I caught Tom in my office lowering the chair as low as it would go. He had done this every day for six months!

As for Jack and Tom, they both retired before they died (Jack was taken from us by that evil cancer thing – there is still time to get even with Tom). With friends and role models like Jack and Tom, how can one go wrong?

Chapter 61

I Think I Love Rachel Ray

"EVOO, Extra Virgin Olive Oil."
- Rachel Ray
(Why does she always use the acronym
and tell us what it stands for?)

September 21, 2003

Update #24. This week was relatively uneventful. It's surprising how long the effects of the chemotherapy drugs wear on and on. By mid week, the worst of the 5-FU had peaked and I finally started to turn the corner. By this weekend, I felt like a real person again (real but another five pounds lighter). I keep up this weight loss and I'll look like a POW. Laura reminds me that I weighed less than this at our wedding. My only comeback is – "Yeah, but look at those pictures!" I need to EAT! Watching the food channel does not equate to eating. (I do have a crush on that 30-minute chef lady, Rachel Ray – I think Ben dumped JLo to date her).

I finally found a personal use for these updates. As I struggled through the week, I went back and read the updates from the previous month to "remember" how soon this week would end. It was surprising how repeatable the effects were – these updates might actually be useful next month too. This was the duplicate week of the "every symptom is associated with a new cancer" week. The difference this time is the mental relief from the clear MRI. It continues to surprise Laura and me how slow I seem to be in responding to these chemotherapy drugs. The pattern repeats but it sure does drag. Good news – only one more time! Bad news – one more time!

News on the work plan – Doctor signed paperwork for me to start work on the 20th – of OCTOBER! Not exactly what I had in mind but I'll make it work somehow. A year from now I'll wonder why I was in such a rush to get back to the grind. From my current *perspective, grinding would be a blast and a sure sign that I'm gonna make it. October 20th will come soon enough.*

My kids want to try to get a count of the number of people who receive (and read) these updates. If you get this email (and read down this far) please send a reply to: cacarters07@comcast.net

If you don't read this far down before you hit delete then feel free to request being deleted from the mailing list. Good luck!

Until next week, I hope your life is as good as mine. I continue to be blessed with the greatest things in life – family, friends, and now – my health. That light is getting brighter and I don't hear a horn.

Love, Mike

Chapter 62

Apple Road

"Nobody goes there anymore, it's too crowded."
- Yogi Berra

Once upon a time in a far away land, there was a boy named Al. Al and Mike were on Christmas vacation (for historical accuracy and anyone investigating the authenticity of Al stories – it was December 31, 1975). They decided they wanted to go see their Biology teacher, Mrs. Oliver. Mrs. Oliver was on maternity leave and hadn't been at school since the previous school year. Mrs. Oliver was also very, very cute and one of their favorite teachers. Mrs. Oliver lived on Apple Road just north of Clough Pike in Clermont County. Luckily, Mike had a map of Clermont County published by the county engineer's office. Mike and Al knew the map would be up-to-date and accurate since Mike's Uncle Walt was the county engineer. Mike and Al looked at the map and realized that there was a shortcut from Al's house to Mrs. Oliver's. All they had to do was pick up Apple Road in Amelia, cut across to Clough Pike and find the new Apple road extension just a few blocks down the road. So, off they went, in Al's Dad's car.

Apple Road leaving Amelia was a beautiful road. It was lined with nice houses, green grass, shade trees, children playing, and dogs barking. Pretty soon, we noticed that the road was a little narrower, there weren't as many houses, green grass, children playing, or dogs barking. There were more trees. As Mike and Al went further they noticed that there weren't hardly any houses, or grass, or dogs barking or children playing. The road had turned to gravel and all they could see were trees. A little further and there were no houses or grass, or children playing or dogs barking. There was just a dirt road and lots and lots of trees. Pretty soon Apple Road was hardly a road at all, it was more like two ruts heading down a steep hill. Mike and Al knew - Apple Road went through on the map - so down they went. Down, down, down. It was a long way down. PLOP.

At the bottom of the hill, Mike and Al were sitting in the middle of the world's largest mud puddle. So they revved and revved and revved. No luck. So they revved forward and backward and forward and backward. No luck. Al finally decided one of them had to get out and push. Al handed the wheel over to Mike and out he jumped, into the mud. So Al pushed and Mike revved, Al pushed and Mike revved, Al pushed and Mike revved (too hard) and Mike splattered Al with mud from head to tow. Still – no luck. Al said, "We're stuck." So out they both jumped. Now, Mike was muddy too but nothing like Al.

Al decided he had to go and get help so he hiked back up the hill to the nearest house (not as close as you would think, for a road that goes through on the map.) Al called a tow truck. Mike and Al met the driver at the top of the hill, just where the road changed from gravel to dirt (right at about the last house). The driver asked them, "Where's your car boys?"

"Down at the bottom of the hill, stuck in a mud puddle," Al answered.

"This ain't no road boys," he said.

"It goes through on the map!" Al answered.

"You boys need to think when you drive," he said.

"I ain't taking my tow truck down there, I'll get stuck too. I'm out of here." And off he drove.

Al decided he had no choice. He had to call his Dad. When Al's Dad arrived Mike and Al met him at the top of the hill just where the road changes from gravel to dirt (right at about the last house). Al's Dad asked, "Where's my car boys?"

"Down at the bottom of the hill, stuck in a mud puddle,," Al answered.

"This isn't a road boys," he said.

"It goes through on the map!" Al answered.

"Al, you need to think when you drive," he said.

They all walked down the hill, took one look at Al's Dad's car and noticed that Al's Dad was just standing there, shaking his head. They all walked back up to the top of the hill to the car that wasn't stuck in the mud puddle, got in, and they drove home. The whole time, Al's Dad never said a word. As Mike jumped out of the car at home, Al whispered, "I'll call you."

In the mean time, Mike was late for a babysitting job. Mike was supposed to watch his cousin Susan while his aunts and uncles went to the Maisonette for dinner. Mike was in trouble on multiple fronts, but nothing like Al. Al called that night and said, "I have a plan," (always dangerous). "Pick me up at my house at 11:30 tomorrow, we have to be at the top of the hill at high noon."

They arrived at the top of the hill just before noon and Al still wouldn't tell Mike the plan. Soon, up rolls a big tractor from Gray's towing. The driver asked them, "Where's your car boys?"

"Down at the bottom of the hill, stuck the mud," Al answered.

"This ain't no road boys," he said.

"It goes through on the map!" Al answered.

"You boys need to think when you drive," he said. "Hop on!"

So down the hill they went. At the bottom of the hill, there was the car, settled even deeper in the mud than last night. The driver handed Al the hook, Al waded in and hooked onto the axel. The tractor pulled Al's Dad's car right out of the mud and all the way to the top of the hill. Fifty dollars later, they were off to Mrs. Oliver's house with one of the best Al stories of all time.

Uncle Walt, when asked about the accuracy of the Clermont County Map said, "Hell, that road hasn't gone through in 50 years, everyone knows that." He was right – everyone does know it now.

Chapter 63

2.5×10^1

"When someone asks you if you're a god, you say 'yes!'"
- Winston Zeddemore, Ghostbusters

September 28, 2003

Update number 2.5×10^1. After all the font troubles I've had, using scientific notation is always a risk. But after a good week like this last one, taking risk feels good. This has been a very good week. I keep thinking, if I feel this good after the last treatments, I can handle it.

I've begun to exercise regularly, walking almost twenty-five miles this last week. We were a little concerned that this would contribute to my weight loss, but the increase in activity was offset by an increase in eating and I gained four pounds this week. Can't do that too many weeks in a row but for now, I'm just eating everything I can. The addition of a daily milkshake seems to be right on the mark.

The responses to last weeks' request for a count of the number of readers are in. We had a total of 227 email responses with many commenting that there were multiple readers in each household. Winner of the First Response Award is Steve Landry of Baltimore, MD. Steve, we thought you had a life. Responding at 10:57pm Pacific Time from Baltimore (2:57 am) is a counter-indicator. I especially enjoyed hearing from people I don't know. My Aunt Sara wins the title of "most notes forwarded to strangers." It's a strange way to make new friends, but it sure makes one feel good. All but one recipient knew, at least in principle, who I was. This one last guy wrote, "I get your update but I have no idea who you are. I wish you well but can you take me off your distribution list?" Oh well, only one complaint – he's been spammed!

I've decided to come clean and I'm working toward full disclosure on my long list of side effects. The one side effect I've been keeping secret is now "out in the open" so I guess I should warn everyone. Ever since the surgery, radiation, and chemotherapy began, I've been plagued with a most embarrassing side effect. Somehow, my normal routine for getting dressed has changed (or my mind is going) and I routinely fail to zip up my zipper. Yeah – not pretty. Laura thinks I should reassess the side effects nicknames, swapping the name of the hiccups (little Ricky). I don't think that's funny. Unfortunately, I'm out of I Love Lucy characters. If I knew there were this many side effects I would have chosen the Brady Bunch. I could call this new one "Marcia, Marcia, Marcia!"

The doctor's office called to remind me to get a blood test before I came in for my chemotherapy this Monday. I said, "WHEN?" They said, "the 28th." I said, "I don't think so." Well, they are full on the 6th and couldn't get me in. I tried to talk the nurse into just canceling me and calling it done, but she didn't fall for that. I'm now scheduled for the 7th. One day's delay works for me. I should have a slightly more relaxing weekend coming up.

The week ahead looks like it will be another good one. I have big plans this week including – filling up the cars with gas, eating, trying a new milk shake flavor, walking the streets of my neighborhood (after checking for Marcia, Marcia, Marcia) and, if all goes well, soaking a few hooks in the mountains. Laura says I'm pushing it too hard. So be it. That loveable, obsessive-compulsive nature is coming back.

The family is still doing great. Dave went to his first dance and has now danced with more girls in his life than I have. Sarah bought a formal dress for homecoming. She's her Aunt Lynn's girl - finding a $121 dress for $17. She's going to look great.

I'll close for now and leave you with one thought – it'll be a great day when these weekly updates end. That day is coming soon – get the fork ready. I'm almost done.

Love, Mike

Chapter 64

Poor Timmy

"They've had a basic medical training, yes."
- Bad wicked, naughty Zoot, Monty Python and the Holy Grail

When Laura and I first enrolled our kids in the Lawrence Livermore National Lab daycare program, our friend Ellen Tarwater-Clower and I met with Kathy Graber (the head of the after-school program for elementary school children of Lab employees) for the mandatory orientation. She told us one of my favorite stories of all time, and it's supposedly true.

A few months prior to our enrollment, the daycare had an incident on the playground. Timmy, a kindergartener, was playing on the monkey bars when slipped and fell and ended up high in the air with a metal crossbar stuck between his legs. Timmy had let out a blood-curdling scream. The teachers ran to his aide, got him down from atop the monkey bars, and tried to figure out what had happened and how badly he was hurt. Timmy was holding his crotch, like all injured males do, and kept saying weakly, "I think I'm bleeding. I think I'm bleeding."

The daycare staff had just finished a daylong training course in sexual abuse awareness to learn to spot signs of sexual abuse in the home. This class also taught the staff how to protect themselves from accusations of sexual abuse in the workplace. Time to put the training to use. This was not a drill.

The all-female staff ushered Timmy to the restroom with instructions for Timmy to go into the restroom and check to see if he was bleeding. Timmy was in the restroom for a few minutes and all they heard through the door were Timmy's moans.

They quickly decided, they needed to go in. As taught in the training classes, Kathy and another female teacher went in together to check on poor Timmy.

They found Timmy standing in the center of the restroom, holding his crotch repeating, "I think I'm bleeding." So they approached Timmy, Kathy down on one knee. They asked Timmy to unbuckle his belt, undo his pants and drop his pants so that they could see if he was ok. Timmy complied and upon closer inspection, they found no blood.

Kathy looked up and asked Timmy, "Are you ok?"

He repeated, "I think I'm bleeding."

Kathy responded from her knees, "Where?"

With his pants down around his ankles, Timmy reached up, pulled down his lower lip and said, "Right here."

Kathy said to the other teacher, "We're dead."

Chapter 65

Smith and Wesson

"If you live long enough, you will be killed by an elephant."
  - Bob Tarwater

October 5, 2003

Update #26. After last week's update revealing my problems with the Brady Bunch, I'm not sure I have much to add. No interaction with the medical community this week – yeah! I put another twenty-five miles behind me this week and find myself at my weight before the last chemotherapy treatment in September. This is the first time I have successfully gained all the weight back before the next treatment (I think that's a good sign). It certainly is a good indicator for the long-term.

This last week, I continued to explore my food options ranging from the medium-rare, USDA Choice, grilled rib eye steak to the McDonald's hamburger. Guess which one hit the spot. I discovered a new steak sauce made by Smith and Wollensky (Smith and Wollensky is a "famous" steak house better known as Smith and Wesson – the prices are so high, you feel like you've been robbed at gunpoint). How do I know that this is the best steak sauce on the market? – Well – It's the most expensive! People wouldn't pay that much for it if it weren't the best! (Same as my wine buying theories). The economy needs consumers like me.

The family spent this last weekend at a friend's cabin in the mountains. It's a fantastic place to go and get away from the television. The four of us played euchre for hours both Friday and Saturday night. Friday night was a blast – I played the entire night and didn't call trump once. My in-laws would have disowned me. On Saturday, we took one of those "let's over do it" family hikes through the giant sequoias. I recovered by sleeping two hours in the late afternoon. They recovered by sitting and reminding me that I over did it. Hey! It's my personality shining through! Five miles at five thousand feet – we should be able to do that without a nap.

I did get out fishing this week. We took the kids to the Stanislaus River. I've decided that the best place to fish in California is Safeway. The fish bite just as well as in the rivers and they are easier to catch. They also come cleaned and filleted.

After this last weekend away, the kids actually suggested we take one night every week and make a TV-free night. Sounds great but I need my "Whose line is it anyway?" fix. I'm as bad as the kids are.

After last week's reference to my Aunt Sara, I've been asked to write a clarification. I'm not sure how my comments got miss-interpreted but my Aunt Sara is almost younger than me. The key word there is "almost." She's been "almost" younger than me for my whole life (and for all but the first six years of hers). I'll add that, when I was born, she wanted me to be a girl! Oh well – she lost that one too. Now she's stuck with me for the duration.

We're working on our list of questions for the oncologist as we enter this final stretch. What's the follow-up plan? When will you do the next CAT scan, MRI, PET scan, etc.? What's the prognosis on the salivary glands? Why do I have to deal with Marcia, Marcia, Marcia? When should I have the feeding tube removed? Let's work out a longer-term back-to-work plan. What are my odds of being killed by an elephant? Lots to talk about. I bet he dreads our appointments as much as we do. I go back to the surgeon in about two weeks. He will likely scope my throat and refer me to physical therapy. I hate being scoped! I think I'll make him make eye contact with me – that'll make it even.

I'll close for now and finish getting ready for the next two weeks. It's only two more weeks and then (I think) I'll be done (or finished)! As my personal philosopher, Bob Tarwater, tells me: "If you live long enough, you will be killed by an elephant." Wish me luck!

Love, Mike

Chapter 66

Stuck

"Hope is the worst of evils, for it prolongs the torments of man."
- Friedrich Wilhelm Nietzsche

There are so many stories from the days in the nuclear test program at the Nevada Test Site (NTS) that one never knows where to start. It's a close-knit group of people that have worked nuclear tests at NTS. We all share a common bond – conquering the elements, conquering the isolation, conquering nature, getting the data and conquering the nuclear designers. One story rises to the top, illustrating the adventure, comradery, and the nature of the humor found with a bunch of geeks in isolation in the middle of the Nevada desert.

Once upon a time, in a far away land, one of my colleagues, Jim Hall was doing a shot. He too was an experimentalist and adventurer by nature. Jim had a free afternoon and decided to explore 40-mile canyon, a remote, isolated area on the western edge of the NTS just north of Area 27. 40-mile canyon had no paved roadway (not unusual for remote areas of the test site). It was just a desert wash canyon and a great area to explore. Jim headed up the canyon in his government car (probably a Ford Fairlane if Pat - the car witch at the Test Site - had anything to do with it) equipped only with a two-way radio tuned to net six, a spare tire, and a jack.

A few miles up the canyon, Jim got his precious government car stuck on a big rock in the middle of the dry wash. Having tried everything in his power to get free, Jim turned to the radio for help. The NTS radio network consisted of multiple channels, many repeaters and continuous monitoring by everyone at NTS and security and safety officials at the control point (CP). Jim explained his predicament and asked politely for help. Well, 40-mile canyon, along the far west edge of the Test Site, is a long way from everything – not to mention – no one ever went anywhere near it.

After getting some useless advice from miscellaneous persons, a fellow Livermore veteran, Jack Morton, came over the radio (net six) and suggested, "Jim, have you thought of just jacking it off?"

Jim Hall replied in the ever-calm voice, "Well, that might make me feel better but I'm not sure it would help me get the car out."

Maybe you just had to be there…

Chapter 67

A Drought of Biblical Proportions

"Someday, you will complain about dry mouth."
- Dr. Jansen

"I don't think so."
- Me

October 13, 2003

Update #27. Well, now I know why they had been giving me chemotherapy on Mondays. When they slip a day, the state of mind for the Sunday night update is just not there yet. I think I set the record for most hours slept in a weekend. Beat my old college records by a landslide.

The good news: They are now officially done dumping chemo drugs into me. The bad news: I'm not done dumping it out yet. There is just nothing you can do to make the drugs flush through any faster. It just has to run its course. As of this morning, I'm pretty much past the cisplatin effects and revving up for the sore mouth from the 5-FU. Just a few more days of misery and then we're back and running again.

The oncologist says my prognosis is excellent – for returning to wine drinking "in moderation." He tells me that this nasopharynx cancer is not related to smoking and excessive drinking of expensive wines. He doesn't tell me what it is related to (see the southeast Asian male comments below). We have a follow-up plan: get an MRI scan once every three months for the first two years and keep our eye out for anything else odd – what ever that means. He says recurrence is most likely local and within the first two years. More optimistically, we have this beat but we'll keep our eyes on it. I do have a few things to watch for – facial twitching, weight loss, throat pain, annoying coworkers, bad vintages.

We just returned from the radiation oncologist. Nice guy, Dr. Chinn. He takes credit for getting the tumor in the parapharyngeal space – gives blame to the surgeon and oncologist for all the other side effects. Again, the prognosis is good but not out of the woods for the next few years. He too has no idea of the cause (unless I'm a Southeast Asian Male with an excess of salted fish in my diet). Close, but – I'm a little short on the salted fish. All the doctors say – return to normal as much as you can – get some strength back by eating and exercising. In the long term, eat a balanced diet (including wine and sushi). And be sure to go to the dentist regularly. Apparently, even a small reduction in salivary function can have disastrous long-term effects on your teeth. What I have is a far cry from "small reduction" – more like a drought of biblical proportions.

All in all, I guess I'm doing better than Rush Limbaugh, although I have some leftover morphine I'll send him in exchange for an autograph. This time next week – I'll be living in the fast lane again! We're almost there!

Love, Mike

Chapter 68

Lawn Care

"We're just negotiating price."
- Sir Winston Churchill

There were many interesting characters at the Nevada Test Site. One of the technicians working for EG&G at the time was Al Martinez. Al was Hispanic, had a very good paying job as a mechanical technician at the Nevada Test Site, and lived in a very nice neighborhood on the northwest side of Las Vegas. One Saturday, Al was working on his lawn in front of his house. Al was down on all fours trimming the edge of the grass along the sidewalk.

A lady in a pink Cadillac pulled up along Al, rolled down her passenger-side window and asked Al, "How much do you charge to do lawns?"

Al replied, "The lady here lets me sleep with her."

The lady rolled up the window and sped off.

Chapter 69

5-FU Sucks!

"They don't call it 5-FU for nothing."
- Kaiser Chemotherapy Nurse

October 19, 2003

Update #28. Now I remember... 5-FU sucks! The oncologist tells me "People complain about the Cisplatin but not the 5-FU." The chemotherapy nurses say – it's the second week that the 5-FU catches up with you. And, true to form (just like the last two months) – the nurses are right again. I figured it out finally – no one makes doctor's appointments the week after chemotherapy – only the nurses hear the complaints. To review: 5-FU sucks the life from you. I spent two days this week in the chair staring at myself wondering if I would ever eat again. All that weight I had gained last month – GONE in three days. The knowledgeable reader will point out the high likelihood of dehydration – Thanks for the help. I had forgotten again how that second week drags on and on.

Well, it's finally behind me. For the record – the 5-FU only lasts a few minutes in the bloodstream but a week or so after you take it, your mouth/throat/digestive system lining finishes the dying process (hopefully killing any remaining cancerous cells preferentially). This makes for an incredibly difficult eating process. Somehow, it's worse than the Cisplatin. At least with the Cisplatin, you don't have enough energy to stay awake.

I'm wondering, is it "all down hill from here?" - easy sailing? Is the hard fight behind me? Or is it "All uphill from here?" Have I hit rock bottom and now it's the climb back to good health? I don't know whether it's uphill or downhill from here but it sure is nice to be here.

Laura and I finally resumed walking at the end of the week. I had gone a few days just sitting in the chair thinking about getting up and getting some fluids in me. You can spend a lot of time thinking about the same "trivial" thing over and over without having the energy to act on it. Again this month – I probably should have gone in for an IV to get my fluid levels back up. But I didn't have the energy to think of that.

By weeks end, I was doing my Emeril imitation (the cooking not the corny acting stuff he does). My biggest challenge – how to get my two new cast iron Dutch ovens in our little oven at the same time. If anyone noticed a drop in the western power grid Friday evening – we were cooking with the oven door partially open. At least PG&E loves me.

By the way – this has been a great week. Sarah (our Freshman daughter) successfully got herself and her ten closest friends through their first homecoming dance – without a single guy. This was not just a dance – it was the Freshman Girl Event of the Year (so far). The first friend arrived on Friday afternoon to begin to get ready.

Saturday morning at 10 am it really got started. By 4:30 on Saturday afternoon, we had ten high school girls all doing the hair/makeup/nails/dress/shoes thing. Dinner for twelve at Chevy's was at 5:00. By 6:30 they were all back at our house doing "touch-ups." As we drove to the dance, I overheard one of them say, "It seems like it's already over." They put so much energy into getting ready that the dance was almost an afterthought. They all looked great and had a wonderful time – guy free.

Weekends like this one make it all worthwhile. I can't wait till the next "event."

This week, I begin a new stage in life – Work! Not quite sure I remember what to do so, if anyone has any life skills tips, I'm up for a good laugh. I also get to visit the friendly, neighborhood head and neck surgeon this week. I have some issues with what he is planning to do to me. I'd love to tell him "NO!" but I'd better just tough it out one more time.

Love, Mike

Chapter 70

Jimmy

"What smell?"
- John "Juan" Hernandez

Work at the Nevada Test site was filled with hazards. We typically worked in the "forward area" up on Piute Mesa about an hour north of Mercury Nevada. The process of preparing the diagnostics to measure the output of an underground nuclear was time consuming. It started with building a canister to hold the nuclear device and installing diagnostic lines of sight and nuclear detectors to record the time history of the nuclear explosion. We had pioneered the use of optical streak cameras to record signals downhole. This diagnostic breakthrough had enabled high time resolution measurements with thousands of channels of data simultaneously. The process of getting the streak cameras calibrated, timed and ready would take a few months of work at the top of a ten-story tower erected on the top of the mesa an hour from the closest "civilization," Mercury, Nevada.

We spent many long days with our streak cameras at the top of the canister in relative isolation from other work going on lower in the tower. On one particular shot, the nuclear device and its' surroundings were particularly sensitive and the plan was to purge the bottom of the canister with ammonia after the device was delivered to ensure there was no possibility of environmental contamination. This system needed to be tested before the nuclear device was delivered.

Warnings were issued throughout the tower alerting us to the possibility of an ammonia leak that might force an evacuation down the 10-story spiral staircase. We often had spiral staircase races (up and down) so a rapid evacuation was not only possible but also something we "practiced." We were warned to be aware of either an emergency announcement or the smell of ammonia. (I wasn't sure I knew exactly what that smell was but I was ready).

My colleagues (and "friends") on the 10th floor of the tower that day were: John Scarafiotti (Scarf), John Hernandez (Juan), and Jimmy Jackson. I put "friends" in quotes for a reason.

Come mid-morning we were working away and I'd hear the occasional "sniff, sniff" from one of the trio. At one point, John Hernandez was heard saying "Sniff, sniff. Scarf, do you smell something?" Scarf's response ("no") put me back at ease.

A little later, I heard all three of them sniffing and whispering to each other, "You guys smell ammonia?" "I don't know." "Smells kind of funny."

I sniffed and ask the Johns "I don't smell anything. What does ammonia smell like?"

"You'll know it when you smell it." Was the reply from Scarf.

A little later, another "Sniff, Sniff" behind me.

I still didn't smell anything. Maybe I wasn't sensitive to the ammonia they were smelling. This was not very comforting. Ammonia was dangerous.

I turned around just as Jimmy was sniffing loudly and watched him fall, face first, on the plywood floor of the 10th floor of the tower.

I leapt from my chair and made a beeline for the corner of the tower and the spiral staircase escape route. As I got to the top of the stairs I looked back to see the trio standing and laughing their heads off… they had set me up.

Now they really knew how much help I would be in the event of a real emergency.

Chapter 71

So Long Brown Cow

"Don't do anything you enjoy during your chemo week."
  - Kaiser Chemotherapy Nurse

October 26, 2003

Update #29. This week was much better than last. The effects of the 5-FU are pretty much behind me and now it's just a slow steady recovery. This week brought a trip to the surgeon (see paragraph below) and a return to work (part time). Things are definitely on the up swing. The big question now is – how many more weekly updates can I write without boring the audience. I may have to start making stuff up.

In response to many emails encouraging me to do something with the evolving story, we have begun to populate a web site with the weekly updates and other family stories and pictures. Please feel free to visit and comment on how I could make it better. Once I write an intro page and write an "update prequel" covering the diagnosis and surgery phases, I will contact the head and neck cancer support groups on line and see if they will put in a link to my site. I know in the early days of my treatments I read a lot of the stories on line and, in general, I found them informative and useful (although void of any humor). I may have to improvise a few details from April but that's not all that different than this update.

You will note the title of the web site is Carters Way. Laura and I had a big debate (argument) about the use, or non-use of an apostrophe. She notes that I always get my way (so add the apostrophe). I think of it as the equivalent to Carters Lane. Hey – at least we're arguing about something important.

I'm eating as well as I have anytime since April. I even recovered from an early mistake. The chemotherapy nurses warn you NOT to eat your favorite foods during the weeks after your chemotherapy treatments. They point out that nausea can spoil your future appetite for that favorite food (if you know what I mean). Did I listen? – NO! One of my favorites WAS – Brown Cow Yogurt (made from whole milk and extra sugar). Well, just after my first chemotherapy I was forced to taste the Brown Cow twice (it was much better going down) and have not wanted to go near it since. I had my first post-chemotherapy Brown Cow this week and it was good – but only tasted it once!

Returning to work this week was a real treat. I can't tell you how nice it is to get back and interact with the people at the lab. Working two hours a day is not as easy as it sounds. Getting out after only two hours is extremely difficult. I did reasonably well avoiding exhaustion but I have a ways to go before those ten to twelve hour days. I'll ask for a cot in my office just in case.

I visited the surgeon on Thursday. Dr. Jansen did what all good doctors do – blame the side effects on someone else. This visit he chose the radiation oncologist. He tells me that my mouth and throat look clear. There is still some tissue swelling and swelling of the spinal column from the radiation treatments. This is apparently the cause of most of my side effects at this point (the neuropathy and the lack of circulation in the extremities). He says the swelling will subside over the next year and a half. A year and a half? I guess that radiation is worse than I thought. I'm beginning to understand the 40 gray (400 rad) lifetime dose limit for the spinal column. Dr. Jansen wants to scope me once a month for the foreseeable future. He obviously enjoys it more than I do. They are watching mainly for a local recurrence. Dr. Jansen says that's unlikely to kill me (partly because it's easier to detect). The more dangerous recurrence is most likely metastasis to the lungs. They will watch for that with chest x-rays and CAT scans over the next two to three years. I'm still rooting to be killed by the elephant (I'm also keeping away from zoos and circuses for the obvious reasons).

All in all – this was a great week.

Love, Mike

Chapter 72

Education by Multiple Means

"He told me that his teachers reported that . . . he was mentally slow, unsociable, and adrift forever in his foolish dreams."
- Hans Albert Einstein, on his father, Albert Einstein

Once upon a time in a far away land, there was an evil math teacher named Mrs. Quinlan. Her evil was not universally accepted but was clearly recognized by the intellectually superior students in the school. Year after year, Quinlan was voted "most popular teacher" – what were those jocks thinking? Quinlan loved the jocks and hated the nerds. I guess we just didn't have enough nerds to stage an effective rebellion. Anyhow, I had Quinlan for calculus during my senior year in high school. I sat next to one of my best friends and fellow nerd, Steve Justice. Even at this young age, Steve was clearly intellectually superior to everyone in the school including the teachers, principal, school board, and superintendent (his father). Steve and I both detested Quinlan for her attitude, intellect, teaching approach and knowledge of calculus.

One day, about halfway through first semester, I asked a question (a question that turned out to be a stupid question I'm sure but – hey it's my first time through calculus). Quinlan stood in front of the class; her arms crossed with a disgusted look on her face and just stared back at me. She just stared and stared and stared in dead silence. It seemed like a minute. The silence was finally broken by Steve Justice's comment just loud enough for the class and Mrs. Quinlan to hear "Education by intimidation."

Steve could have done anything he wanted in life. His experience with Mrs. Quinlan clinched the deal. Steve dropped calculus after the 1st semester. Steve went on to become a professor in Medieval Literature at the University of California at Berkeley. I went on to get a D in calculus my senior year even though the cheerleaders and football players probably ended up with B's or even A's. To this day, when I drive past Quinlan's house I ask if anyone has a dozen eggs... I don't plan on cooking breakfast... except maybe on the hood of her car.

Steve Justice is famous for another great one liner in calculus class. Steve was the son of the superintendent of the school district, Fleming Justice. Straight laced, conservative, smart as anyone you've ever met and a classic nerd (except for his exceptional mastery of the alto sax). We're sitting in calculus class one day, taking a quiz or test. The entire room was quiet except for the scribbling of the #2 pencils on the paper (or the groans of the football players – or whatever noise they make when they know they don't know shit but will get an A in a class from the "teacher of the year" every damn year – I still hate her 30 years later). So breaking the silence was Steve's classic one liner. That's right – Steve Justice.

"*Fuck!*"

Now that was not what we were expecting...

Steve was sent to the office where they promptly sent him back to class. They didn't believe the story either.

Chapter 73

Bye Bye Feeding Tube

"You only require two things in life: your sanity and your wife."
- Tony Blair

November 2003

Monthly Update #1. Welcome to the first edition of the Carter Monthly update. For those of you used to the weekly fix – feel free to reread this update 4 times. You can even forward it to yourself each week so it looks like a new email. This last week was better than ever. I am continuing to gain weight (at a rate I can't sustain for long). My strength and stamina are also continuing to improve.

We celebrated Laura's birthday last Wednesday. The kids and I took Laura to Wente's restaurant (the best restaurant in the Livermore valley). The kids got all dressed up and surprised Laura when she got home from work. We had a really nice time. It's great to see the kids growing up and able to act it for a few continuous hours.

Thursday afternoon saw me trek to Napa in search of great wine for my winter ski trip to Colorado. Every year it's the same challenge – can you drink great wines and ski in the same week? I sure am glad I didn't lose my sense of taste during the radiation and chemotherapy. The oncologist says – drink in moderation is ok (alcohol is not a big risk factor for this cancer). His definition of moderation and mine may differ slightly. Anything has to be better for you than dumping chemo drugs into your veins.

Friday night was Halloween. Making fun of Mom and Dad, Sarah went as a girl from the 70s (bell bottoms, 70s blouse, and peace sign). Dave went as a man in his pajamas. The candy haul was impressive. Now we're picking up candy wrappers for the next few weeks (or days if their rate continues).

This weekend brought back some great memories. We went to see the local musical company's production of West Side Story. It was wonderful. Sarah was not that happy with the way it ends (three dead guys). I had played in the orchestra when we did West Side Story in high school so it brought back many great memories. (I cried through the whole thing.) Yeah – I'm weak...

I finally had my feeding tube removed this morning (Tuesday November 4). This is an interesting procedure. The GI doctor stands in the procedure room (right near the door for a quick get away if anything starts to go wrong). The nurse dresses in a "space-suit-like" gown complete with full-face shield. They have you lying flat on the table with the nurse leaning over you (hey it's not all bad). She puts one hand on your stomach and wraps the tube around the other hand and she pulls (more like yanks). The tube just pops right out – hurts much less than they had warned me. Apparently the space-suit getup is not a holdover from Halloween but a splashguard. They slap on a Band-Aid and send you on your way. They ask you to take only water for the first four hours. Apparently, the stomach heals much faster than one would think. You can return to eating by dinnertime. So far – so good. The doctor didn't faint either.

Well – I'd better get this out before I get more email messages from people wondering if they have been dumped from the list...

See you in December for monthly update #2.

Love, Mike

Chapter 74

Al's Suntan

"Go to Heaven for the climate, Hell for the company."
- Mark Twain

Once upon a time in a far away land, there was a boy named Al. Al came home from school one beautiful sunny day and decided he needed a suntan. Al grabbed his favorite book, changed into his swim trunks, found his sunglasses, and set up the lounge chair in the front yard right near the sidewalk where he would be sure to capture every available ray from the sun. Al laid back, put his sunglasses on and began to read. Well, the neighbors drove by, stared and commented "That darn Al" or "look at him now" or "What is Al thinking?" The occasional honk and shout of "get inside" was the only noise that broke the calm.

Al seemed to be the only one not to realize that there was six inches of snow on the ground.

Or maybe he knew...

Chapter 75

Thanksgiving – My Favorite Holiday

"It's a free country."
- Dr. Jansen

December 2003

Monthly Update #2. It's been a while. I think weekly is too frequent but monthly is not quite often enough. A lot has happened in the last month (mostly good stuff). I feel sort of out of touch with my email friends around the country but – monthly will have to do. I'll make it work.

Quick health update: All has gone well during the last five weeks. I think there has only been one trip to the doctor. As I was sitting in the chair being scoped (fiber optic viewer up the nose and down the throat), the surgeon says, "So I hear you've been writing about me." (Remember this is the guy who can carry a conversation only if eye contact can be avoided). I'm thinking – OH, I'm in trouble – He's got me right where he wants me - I've actually used his real name too!!! It turns out; one of my friends on the update list is a recent patient of his and has spilled the beans. I confessed my sins and he says, "Hey – it's a free country, write whatever you want."

This doctor knows I think the world of him (but most surgeons assume that as a starting condition). Somehow, I talk my way out of the chair and escape unharmed. From now on, I'll be more careful to develop a cover story before visiting these guys. I will not refrain from telling doctor stories out of school. By the way, Dr. Jansen says, "pretend you are cured" (actually he says – "behave like you are cured" – subtle difference).

I have not continued to gain weight (I'm actually down a few pounds from my recent high) – It turns out that eating is not one of those tasks you can relegate to the "miscellaneous background activities of life" list. It's become a chore. I want my allowance if it's going to be this hard. I also had the joy of catching a cold from the kids just before thanksgiving. I've decided that my old fat reserve was a nearly endless supply of energy – important when that cold hits – also helps keep you warm in winter. I'm looking into hibernation but haven't found that code number when filling out my weekly time card.

Side effects from the treatment are still alive and well. Biggest pain in the neck is the dry mouth (I promised the surgeon that I would not complain about "a little dry mouth" if he got me through the surgery. He may have won that bet.) The second biggest pain in the neck is the neuropathy and the poor circulation in the extremities. Who needs feeling in the hands anyhow? The radiation oncologist indicated that this would fade after 3 months. The surgeon points out that the oncologist stops seeing me after three months so from his vantage point – it's faded. The third biggest pain in the neck is the pain in the neck. Sure glad the surgery was above the waist.

Thanksgiving is probably my favorite holiday. We had a houseful again this year (23) and I loved every minute of it. I got the kids (9 of them) working all day on Wednesday (cooking, cleaning, decorating, setting the table, printing the menus etc.). There is so much to be thankful for this year – like the surviving taste buds (Oh and friends and family and life in general... blah, blah, blah) Sure wish I could still drool... The drool enhancement medication is not working. Maybe I should take whatever Hugh Heffner takes – little blue diamonds?

Getting back to work has been a real treat. I have more people making sure I limit my time to four hours a day than ever cared if my lunch hour was longer than 45 minutes. What they don't know is that I go to work to rest. I probably should take them off this distribution.

I made it to DC twice since the last update. The reception I received brought tears to my eyes. Next month I'll ask the surgeon if he can plumb the tear ducts into the salivary glands. Then I can cry at every meal. It sure was nice to get back to the center of the universe and begin to understand the future options. Somehow,

Laura and I (and the kids) have to come up with a "plan." We can't even say the "p word" at our house.

I finally got my flu shot. Finally a plus for the numbness in the arms – I didn't feel a thing. There is always a silver lining. The day after I did notice a sore arm. I also have a symmetric sore arm on the right side (no shot on that side). Go figure.

We're heading home for Christmas again this year. Should be great! We'll have Cincinnati Chili, Gray's (and I'll try to sneak in a few White Castle hamburgers – Laura hates it when I eat them – so – I gotta do it!). Looking forward to seeing the family. It's been a tough year on them too. I'm the only one in the family who took six months off work and got paid for it – I think I'll rub that in a bit.

See you next year for monthly update #3. In the mean time – We hope you all have a Merry Christmas and a Happy New Year. Until then, be sure to think of me when you drool or spit – it's the small things that make life special.

Love, Mike

Chapter 76

Friday Night Dinner

"It's Friday, Friday"
- Rebecca Black (sorry...now that song's in your head)

"Friday Night Dinner" has become a tradition that is important to us. It started when the kids were little. Every Friday afternoon after school our kids were allowed to go to the Clower's to hang out (and eat the Clower's junk food). This group of kids from six families became known as the TP bandits. Once a month or so, they would TP one of their own homes (and clean up the mess the next morning). The TP Bandits: Sarah, David, Brendan, Matthew, Fort, Dana, Patrick, Sarah B., Reyer, and Grace would become lifelong friends. We're not really sure how it started but the parents would come pick up the kids on Friday after work and bring something and stay for dinner. When the kids were old enough to drive (and especially when we moved back to California from Virginia), we began to alternate hosting with the Clowers. This became our weekly tradition and to this day is a major motivator to make it through the week.

We have only a few simple rules: Keep your expectations low. If you are an adult (self defined), bring something to share. The host provides a main course (or more). I try to bring homemade cinnamon rolls each week. It's not fancy or formal – it's just relaxing. Every week it's the same drill – we never know exactly how many people might come. We can have a few as a dozen and as many as 30. What's really special about Friday Night Dinner (FND) is the continued participation of the kids. It's now much more than the TP bandits, it's now expanded to their boyfriends and girlfriends, future boyfriends and girlfriends, friends of their friends, a few other couples and even ex-girlfriends and ex-boyfriends.

Sounds wonderful but Friday nights are not without peril. I take this back to a time many years ago when the Clowers got their first dog from the dog guide school dropout list. Lollie was a beautiful, one year old Golden retriever that had flunked out of guide dog school for some reason I don't remember. Maybe it was because she was the not the sharpest bulb on the Christmas tree or the brightest knife in the drawer. There was something about Lollie's personality that grabbed me and I fell in love in the first few minutes.   Laura and I had a deal from when we got married. I had to pick between her and a dog. I could not have both. As I tell Laura now, if she dies first, I'm taking my to her funeral. Not exactly sure of the point here but – the Clower dogs were our dogs (emotionally). Good deal – all the love – none of the mess.

They had Lollie for less than a week and they got the dreaded call; there had been a mistake. Lollie was being recalled. The family that raised her the first year before dog school had first right if she flunked out. They wanted her back. I was the last to find out and I cried for a few days. I never saw Lollie again and didn't get a chance to tell her how much I loved her. This is the "Lollie syndrome" - too quick to fall in love and can never let go.

The Lollie syndrome is not limited to dogs. I have the same "problem" with the kids' boyfriends and girlfriends: Doug, Hope, Christine, Karen, Big Dana, Kaela, Ashley, Melissa, Jamie and the newest entrée's – Dale and Grady. All are either current, ex-, future ex-, or future spouses, of the Friday Night Dinner group. They are always welcome! I hope none of them ever get recalled.

Chapter 77

Johnny Walker Blue

"Go Blue!"
- Michigan and Johnny Walker fans

January 2004

Monthly Update #3. Well, we finally made it to 2004. 2003 was a great year (for those of you who have to choose between great, good and bad). December and the holidays were wonderful as well – in fact, better than ever. December was filled with freedom; freedom from the doctor visits, freedom from crisis, freedom from worry. I did see three doctors over the Christmas holiday but luckily they were family and friends. Just like all doctors, they give their opinions but I DON'T HAVE TO LISTEN.

The visit home to Indiana and Ohio was particularly good this year. On the Carter side we had the annual convergence of my father's family. It's always dangerous getting the Carter males together as the confluence of opinionation is potentially harmful to the environment. Sounds like a reinvigoration of a Bushism. Since my father passed away seven years ago, I've tried to defend his positions. It's not easy to be opinionated, especially when you're wrong but that's the Carter way. Again this year, the Pattersons joined us just like they are family. In fact, they are just like family. It was especially nice this year.

On Christmas day, almost everyone from my mother's side was there: Mom, My famous (and still young) Aunt Sara, Uncle Don and Alison from Washington, Cousins Dr. Nathan and Dr. Jenn (and their daughter Selah) from St. Louis, My Uncle Leonard, Aunt Donna, and sons Jason and AJ from Columbus. Missing and missed were my brother's family (stranded in the cold in Minnesota), my uncle Jack (often misidentified as my identical twin + 12 years) and his family, and my cousin Susan and her "reportedly" spectacular husband (whose wedding I missed during my alleged bout with cancer).

After a grand Christmas dinner prepared by the greatest chef the Carter family has ever seen (guess which famous writer I'm speaking of now), we had a spectacular day capped off with Graeter's ice cream (Oprah's favorite). Rumor has it that they make more flavors than the Black Raspberry Chocolate Chip but I wouldn't know. Hey, if Oprah likes it, it's gotta be good for you.

On Laura's side, once again we successfully got the entire family together in the same place at the same time to celebrate Christmas. This streak will hopefully continue for the foreseeable future – we're certainly not going to break it. Family came to Indiana from Columbus Ohio, South Carolina, and San Diego. We ate, ate and ate. I don't cook at Laura's house – I just eat (no fudge). Indiana weather was quite pleasant this year – much warmer than the basketball team – It's going to be a long cold winter for the Hoosiers.

We did experience some memorable travel moments courtesy of United Airlines. Lost luggage – both ways. Delayed flights are always nice (4 hours on the tarmac at SFO was a delightful way to start the trip)– more time on the plane but not more frequent flyer miles. They should have frequent waiting miles. Canceled flights are fun. Rerouting through Washington Dulles on a flight that was also canceled is special. Eventually we were rerouted back through O'Hare onto our original flight where we had the pleasure of sitting in International Boeing 777 coach seating. Six of our seven bags were also rerouted (I hope they had more leg room than we did). The last one was routed through TSA headquarters to search for sharp cheeses. The airline food was also memorable – Oreo's, chips, and cheese and crackers all make excellent entrees for the salivarily impaired.

I may be spit-challenged to be a little less PC but I can order a salad off the new $10/entrée menu in United's famed coach class. The good news – we made it all the way back and forth and I didn't have to share any of MY frequent flyer miles.

Amazon.com treated us well delivering gifts the day after they were needed. Outpost.com beat that - delivering the week after Christmas. Santa drives one of those brown trucks and works the week after Christmas. We're sure lucky we have great kids. Hard to believe what you can explain with tic-tacs and a deck of cards in their stockings. We also picked up some horse racing tips from Uncle Pete Rose and tips on handling the press from Cousin Bobby Knight. My three boyhood heroes (Pete, Bobby and Woody Hayes) have had their struggles and I'm now paying the price for questionable judgment in my childhood.

Other highlights of the Midwest included: A reunion of Lou, Al, Dale (I mean Mr. Swisher) and DW; 5 trips to Skyline Chili in 6 days (6/6 if it weren't for Christmas); Gray's Cafeteria in Downtown Mooresville Indiana; our annual evening with Laura's High school friend Monica and Dean; an after-dinner run to the Aluminum Room at the White Castle Lounge with Tyler; nursing a fifth of Johnny Walker Blue (thanks Gary); and the highly desired, edible garments courtesy of Pons (soon to marry our niece Emma). Hey Pons – RUN NOW! – it's not too late... We also finished our test and evaluation of the Homeland-security-approved Airzookas. Harmless? I don't think so!

In Summary: I'm feeling great! Homeland Security Alert level back to Yellow! Cold returns to the Midwest. Next MRI scheduled for January 26. Neuropathy expected to fade just before we land a man on Mars. How could life be better?

See you next month for a pre-Valentine's greeting. It could be my last. I'll cover that in more detail next month..."Oh the humanity!"

Looking for travel opportunities come February 14...

Mike

Chapter 78

The finger(s)

"A true friend is one who knows all about you and likes you anyway."
- Christi Mary Warner

I've been known to tell the same story/joke more than once. The story might not be the same the second time but there is typically sufficient similarity that the second telling often receives some "complaint" from the audience. My closest friends have adopted a practice that "works" for them.

This started when Curtis Clower's sister, a special education, teacher was visiting one summer. In her class was a young autistic boy who liked to tell stories. He (too) would tell the same stories over and over again. In an attempt to not offend him and yet not hear the same stories over and over again, Curtis' sister would hold up two fingers, like the peace sign, to let him know that "they liked this story and he had told it before." They could do this without interrupting and without saying a word. He would stop and smile and they would both move on. Sounds like a clever idea, adopted by both the story receiver and teller.

Laura, Curtis, Ellen, and all our kids, decided that this would be a good idea for dealing with Mike. They would routinely "give me the fingers" if I was telling a story for the second, third, or forth time (or more). We would all laugh and sometimes – I would keep going. It is not unusual to be sitting at the dining table, telling a joke or story and (when I would bother to look around) see half dozen or more pairs of fingers letting me know that they had heard a version of this story before. The fingers were always paired with a smile encouraging me to "continue at my own risk." Offending Ellen and her typically quiet "flying monkeys" was to be avoided at all cost. (She has an hourglass, a crystal ball, a broom, and a bicycle with a basket too). I remind Ellen that my true friends know all about me and like me anyway.

Chapter 79

It Doesn't Get Any Better Than This

*"A pessimist sees the difficulty in every opportunity;
an optimist sees the opportunity in every difficulty."*
- Sir Winston Churchill

February 2004

Monthy update #4. January is finally over. No more NFL football. No more MTV strip shows on CBS. No more time off for disabilities. Life is good anyway. This month was more good news on the doctor front. It started with a trip to the surgeon. I fought a monumental traffic jam, successfully found a parking space in the famous "all drivers are morons parking garage," walked up to the counter and proudly announced that I was here to see Dr. Jansen. The nurse looked up at me and asked, "how are you feeling?" There is only one good answer in this situation. Unfortunately I naively said "Great!" She returned with, "well then, you won't get to see the doctor today." Hot tip – whenever they ask you should be able to recite the symptoms from any major disease such as Ebola or Anthrax. A limp or fake cough is a good idea too. Acting macho like "I can beat this cancer on my own" or similar attitude will put you back in traffic in a few weeks.

I successfully negotiated another MRI this month. 75 minutes in the tube with only one complication. They had a lot of trouble finding a vein with blood flow in it to inject me with the Gadolinium. They use enough Gadolinium to trip the metal detector at the airport – give those TSA guys a good challenge. The blood draw people have the same problem. Both arms are blown out from the chemotherapy. This might explain the cold hands and feet too.

By the time I arrived at the airport (after the MRI), the surgeon had read it and called my beeper and my wife. Only my wife answered. Result – still clear. The radiologist agrees. Sounds like I'm home free for another few months. I had told myself that there is no bad news from an MRI. If they find nothing – great. If they find something – great – I'd rather find it sooner than later. A few months after the chemotherapy has ended I feel like I could take another round if I had to. This same phenomena leads to families with two or more children.

I'm still recovering from the chemotherapy and radiation. The neuropathy in the hands and feet leads to challenges like buttoning my shirt and zipping my zipper. That's my story and I'm sticking with it. My lack of balance is now explainable by the reduced nerve sensation from the feet and not any heredity-related issues. This disease stuff is a great way to cover other underlying issues. I'll test the cold hands and feet problem later this month when I venture off to Colorado for my annual ski trip with Ralph and Ron. If I fall remember – it's the neuropathy!

During a recent trip I was challenged to a future marathon (date TBD). In response, I "ran" a 10K last weekend. Actually, after looking up the word "run" in the dictionary I probably did something else like "glopped." The time was not anything I can type in a serious update like this but I can report the 10km is an accurate number. The dictionary definition of "glopp" is "to simulate a run at a significantly slower, almost laughable pace" (Webster's 2005 edition). OK Harry Vantine – you'd better start worrying – I'm gonna glopp a marathon with you someday!

This coming month brings many challenges: My visit to the surgeon later this week, My quarterly visit to the oncologist next week, Tencia's going away party (my former secretary – whoops I almost said "old secretary") and the most dreaded of all holidays – Valentine's day. If I make it through another one alive I'll write a March update. If not – I did NOT take my own life – no matter what the crime scene looks like. Oh the humanity!

I finally got around to writing the prequel to the cancer story (the times before the first update in April of 2003).

Remember – it doesn't get any better than this!

Love, Mike

Chapter 80

I Need Good Administrative Assistance

"Shit Happens!"
- Ancient Greek, Roman, Chinese, Arab, Egyptian, Aztec, Mayan, Hopi, Viking, and Neanderthal Proverb

So – I'm working at the newly formed, Department of Homeland Security as the Chief Scientist for the Plans, Programs and Budget Section of the Science and Technology Directorate and I've got no help. I apparently am the help. We're preparing for a visit from the White House Homeland Security Council and, we'd like to look good. Look good means: Have a well prepared story, be on time, be organized, be concise, be articulate, have prepared printed material to work from and talk to, and – look good. Dr. Parney Albright assigns me to get the story together, get the material in shape, make copies to talk to, be on time and dress well. Not hard. The visitors: David Howe, Senior Director on the Homeland Security Council, and Col. Julie Bentz, his deputy, are coming at 1pm. They'll look good… and so will we.

The story is easy, the material is taking shape, the suit fits and the tie is tied neatly. It's likely a Hickey Freeman suit and Jerry Garcia tie (I don't really remember the tie but that was the thread of choice those days in my income range). It's the production of the photocopies that emerge on the critical path and – I'm not ahead of schedule and not an expert copy maker.

So: Print the first set – It's 10 till 1… I'm on track. Run the first set through the copier making, let's say – six copies. Put paper in copier, press 6, press GO. It's 12:51… lots of time to get this right. As I do this, I realize I need to make a correction to chart thirteen. Easy. Whoops forgot to push the collate button. I'll collate by hand.

Discard old chart thirteen in recycle bin. I like the bin. It's big (I need big). It's blue. It has a key-shaped hole in the lid: A slot with a circular opening at one end of the slot. The slot is for the paper –

hole must be for your hand (or paper wads). I like the blue color too.

Whoops: Paper jam. It's 12:52. I hate paper jams but I'm technical, I can handle it.

Open door. Pull out jammed paper as it runs through the rollers getting toned and dried and whatever else it is that copiers really do. All we know at this point is admin people should be doing this not scientists.

Throw out jammed paper (in the friendly shaped recycle bin). Lots of jammed paper with that toner powder that's not stuck and dried yet to the paper... messy stuff but – doable.

Jam "cleared!" It's 12:55. I still have lots of time.

I realize as I hand collate the pages that, I've thrown a key set of paper into the slotted recycle bin and I've got to go in for it. Hey – the hole at the end of the slot is for the hand not just paper wads. The paper I need must be near the top. In goes my hand. It's 12:56. There's lots of time still.

I fish around and find the paper I need. I grab it. Now – my hand is too big to pull back out of the hole... I've seen this before... 12:57. Plenty of time still... Release hand – drop paper – pull paperless hand out of hole... Observe interesting phenomena... White shirt has rubbed on edge of slot and is now covered with toner. "Look good" is now behind me.

Reach back in – grab paper. Pull hard. Lid comes off recycle bin with arm still sticking through hole. Paper is now free. Toner is everywhere... Lid still hanging from arm. It's 12:58. Time is just about up...

Drop paper... Release fist... pull arm out... inspect toner on shirt... finish collating.

It's 12:59:99. Time is up. Both the story and material look good. I do not...I need administrative assistance... badly.

Chapter 81

Sign of Success

"I was wrong once. I thought I'd made a mistake."
  - Dr. Bill Nexsen

July 2004

Well, it's been a while since the last update and not a lot has changed. Maybe a few things... This morning the four of us boarded a United flight and headed east for a couple of years. The process of leaving our home and friends was (is) painful. Laura and I moved to California in 1981 just two days after we were married. Neither of us had ever flown on an airplane (our first flight was less than a year later – a memorable United flight on a DC-10 into O'Hare) In the last 23 years, things have changed. I was drawn to the lab by the lure of BIG science. The lab represented applied science at it's finest: a great mix of theory, computations and experiment. As an experimentalist, I favored the latter and the lab seemed to excel in big experiments. I have had the opportunity to work with some great experimentalists over the years:

Bill Nexsen in M-Division (his famous quote "I was wrong once, I thought I'd made a mistake") - Bill was always looking to be wrong. I learned from him that being "wrong" was much more interesting than being "right."

Dick Fortner and Mark Eckart: Dick took a chance on a young experimentalist coming out of M-Division – I still owe him. Mark brought more passion to the job at hand than anyone I've ever known. With his infamous vocabulary (Jeff Hockman probably still keeps the Eckartisms on his white board) and famous quotes "noblesse oblige" and "90 miles an hour with your hair on fire," Mark built a team to get the job done with whatever it took. The night of the Contact event in the summer of 1989 was the highlight of my early career. Mark gets it! It's too bad that Greenwater data never came in. Someday, I'll write the book – "Summer of

'89." My badge of honor was Lowell Wood threatening to fire me. This was nothing short of a macroscopic sign of success.

The Three Musketeers (Dave Fields, Charlie Bennett and Mike Carter): The earliest LIFTIRS data over the Labor Day weekend sometime in the early 90s, Long nights overlooking Area 51, Decoding top secret acronyms like SELF, the Blind tests of Mountain Lion, the first flights in the WB-57, responding to the World Trade Center attacks. We loved the debate and comradery. We built a great team. Oh, if I was as smart as Charlie Bennett...

There were many great personal achievements over the last 23 years also: My two kids: Sarah (Contact baby) and David (Greenwater baby). At least I can remember their birth years – all activities were tied to the Nuclear Test program. They are the most wonderful kids I have ever met – I'm proud to be their Dad. Oh – And Laura hasn't killed anyone yet although I think I'm on the short list. She continues to threaten me with a divorce and she pledges to go after all of my United Frequent Flyer miles. I'll give up the kids but not the miles. Looks like the judge will decide.

I can remember some rough times too: getting beat at chess by my six year old son, (Turns out, they think a few moves ahead) getting two batches of flagstone that almost matched, and that cancer thing.

We begin a journey now. We're off to DC for a few years to work Homeland Security. We move into our new home in early July (when the truck arrives) and begin a temporary, new way of life. Laura and I are planning to commute (together). In Livermore, after a three-mile commute, we parked next to each other in the parking lot every day for the last ten years. We'll enjoy the time together debating the constitutionality of including frequent flyer miles as community property. Last time I checked, her name was NOT on my monthly statement.

By far the hardest part is leaving our friends.

We just landed at Dulles and I've just been beat at my own game. Two months ago, Sarah was forced to take the SAT test as a *freshman just to apply to TJ. Coming out of the exam, I had made Sarah an offer: If she scores above 1320 (the average score of all accepted "incoming" sophomores at TJ the previous year, we would take her to any restaurant she wanted on the bay area. If she scores above 1400 – any restaurant in the US. If above 1500 – any restaurant in the world. If 1600 (a perfect score) – she could choose all the lesser prizes plus – I'd buy her a Porsche. (I must have been confident – little did I know I was playing with fire).*

Her scores came back at a solid – 1340 – winning the bay area restaurant of her choice – BUT – I warned her, If I come home from work next Tuesday and ask her "where do you want to go for dinner tonight?" and she says "McDonalds" – That's her choice! Be warned...

Every night for two months, I'd ask her what she wanted for dinner and she'd say "whatever," "your choice," "Don't care"...

We finally land at Dulles airport and begin the taxi to Terminal C – gate C17... She leans over to me and, out of the blue, and says "Wente!" (Wente is the best restaurant in the Livermore Valley)... I love it when I lose...

Let the next adventure begin.

Mike

P.S. Sarah got her acceptance letter to Thomas Jefferson High School (TJ) later that day (in our mailbox at our new home in Virginia). She'll be pushed to her limit but I have confidence that she will rise above all challenges pushing the bar higher that we can see. She'll also be eating at Wente restaurant in the hills south of Livermore sometime in the near future... my treat.

Chapter 82

Wardrobe Malfunction

"Go ahead, Make my day!"
- Harry Callahan and Ronald Reagan

I have trouble with clothing. It's hard to understand but there is something about expensive suits and people from Mt. Carmel, Ohio that don't go together. Look at my Eagle Scout photos, my Grandparents 50th anniversary, my prom photos, my Graduation, my wedding, the list goes on. The footnote – looking at my grandparents' 50th anniversary you will see an indicator of parental abuse or willful neglect. Who chose those plaid pants? Me and Ed? I think not. This was likely a case of felony child abuse but on with the story.

In the scientific community, there is a well known scientific review board that can make or break a great idea. The JASONs were empaneled by the defense department to advise the DoD on specific research and technology initiatives. JASONs stands for July August, September, October, and November – the months they meet. So, I'm up to brief the JASONs in about 1999. It's my first opportunity to brief this group so the pressure is high. They are famous for going after you and once they get started – get some blood in the water and it becomes a feeding frenzy with every shark on the committee after his bite and no one there to preserve humanity.

I'm talking about the science base for some big DoD program (blah, blah, blah, yada, yada, yada). I'm wearing my suit (yeah – my one suit) and just before going up, I realize that I have two significant problems. The cuff on the pant leg has come undone and the cuff is no longer folded up. It's sagging down and my shoe is stepping on it. I look like a geek wearing his only suit to Halloween party but it's worse than that. You know how the zipper of the pants has a fabric flap covering it, well, some seam is coming out up there too and the flap is falling in the breeze. So up

I go, zipper zipped up but flap flapping and shoe stepping on cuff hanging on the floor.

Luckily, I was not the only geek in the place, in fact, I'm certain absolutely no one noticed. If my formulas had been missing a 2pi, I wouldn't be here today but zippers are for someone else to be concerned with.

A few years later (after the infamous Janet Jackson Super Bowl) I experience another humorous wardrobe malfunction. I had been having suit problems since purchasing Hicky Freeman suits at Nordstrom and experiencing a series of questionable workmanship issues. (see the ring story from the cancer prequel) So, I'm at the Clower's, I'm dressed and I'm having simultaneous loose thread challenges. I ask Ellen for help. The first is up on the collar of the suit coat – I need a thread carefully clipped. Ellen grabs a pair of scissors and does the snip. I then ask her for a bigger favor. I have a big ball of loose threads, obstructing the zipping-up of the pants zipper. This clipping must be done carefully and only by Ellen because – "I'm not a threat."

Chapter 83

Vacation? - Check

"There's no place like home."
- Dorothy Gale

April 2, 2005

Two years ago today was a bad day. In the conventional sense, "bad news" and "Bad days" run together. In hindsight, April 2, 2003 was more of a turning point. It was the eve of what I now refer to as "my summer vacation." On April 2, 2003, I finally made it to Dr. Martinez with my much-delayed CAT scan and after a quick glance she scheduled what was to be my first canceled surgery. I recall quickly working through the stages (denial, anger, acceptance...) like Homer Simpson after eating the ill-prepared Blowfish.

I called Laura on my walk back down Pennsylvania Ave. Even at the time, I kind of knew everything would be OK.
Lets go back to the "summer vacation" for a moment. What is the definition of a vacation?
- Paid time off work? (Check).
- Rest and relaxation? (Check).
- People waiting on you hand and foot? (Check).
- Time to spend with friends, family and loved ones? (Check).
- Time to reflect and write about life? (Check).
- Exploring the joys of new foods? (Check).
- Exposure to radiation and developing a nice sunburn? (Check)
- Ionizing radiation? (Maybe not).

Sounds a lot like a vacation to me...

Things are pretty good on the health front. I still make it back to the head and neck surgeon (Dr. Martinez) about once a month. We do the throat inspection thing (the scoping) and it's become "routine." Comfortable? No but it's not as bad as it once was. I'm on a CAT Scan cycle (once every 4-5 months) that keeps me happy and doesn't stress the system too much. So far – I'm clear. I should probably go in for a complete physical. Looking at the treatments I get every month, (they JUST look at the head and throat – not even a weigh-in or a blood pressure check – not even a stethoscope!) I'm convinced they have a single goal. To be sure I die from something else!

The lingering side effects are more and more manageable. The dry mouth limits the foods I can eat. Breads and other dry foods are still major challenges. Soup and I have become good friends. (Oh and Dove Bars...). The diet leaves something to be desired. My weight has held steady for the last 15 months at 158-159. The Doctors would still like to see me put a few pounds on (I assume they care where). "Anywhere" just encourages the Dove Bar habit. It is from the dairy and chocolate food groups. I still remember Dr. Jansen telling me I'd complain about a dry mouth someday. I thought he was NUTS! He was right – it's a real pain but it does appear to be getting slowly better. I still carry water with me wherever I go (with few exceptions). Invariably I choke on something every meal. Sometimes, that something can be as simple as water. It's just not quite right yet.

I'm pretty much used to the neuropathy. As I joke, "It's not really that bad in the first 4 extremities." Itches that are tough to scratch and no sensation of hunger (or full stomach) are the typical nagging issues that I can speak of in public. The neck is still stiff and sore – That looks like a lifelong condition. The nerve sensation in the neck and shoulder will not return (as promised). The good news is, I'm complaining about the little things. The big things are good – Still have a pulse, able to fog a mirror, continuing to increase the entropy in the universe, can recognize myself in a lineup, babes still think I'm hot, self awareness is still for others. Life is good.

Back at the end of January, David and I joined my brother Ed in Colorado and skied for 3 days at Copper Mountain. A dry mouth and neuropathy are no match for a nice groomed blue run. Strap the boots on tight and pack water in the camelback. The neuropathy just makes you more resilient to the cold. Dave is beyond me, skiing his first black run.

Life in DC is fine. Life in DC is fine. Life in DC is fine. (Dorothy Gale is my role model – she kept saying it and ended up back in Kansas.) This is not the place to talk about work and the struggles of the Washington bureaucracy so, I won't. Life is good and full of good people.

Sarah is thriving at Thomas Jefferson High School for Science and Technology. She wrote a paper on the cancer drug Cisplatin last fall. It was the best treatment of the complexities of Cisplatin on cancer cells that I had read. Chemotherapy is complicated but Sarah made it understandable like no doctor I had talked with. She was asked to submit her paper to the DuPont challenge (which we did – one day late). She didn't win but we're proud. I need to get another cool disease for next year's contest.

Love, Mike

Chapter 84

The Black Mark of Death

"You shall not have been mortally wounded in vain."
- Sir Lancelot, Monty Python and the Holy Grail

I'm coming up on my 5th anniversary of my cancer diagnosis and life throws ever-changing curves. My cholesterol is up (greater than 275), my blood pressure is rising (150s over 110s) and I finally decide, with significant prodding from my administrative assistant, Amy Brooks, to go to the doctor and get a good looking at. Drugs are good – so, they start me on a chemically enhanced, cholesterol lowering, blood pressure lowering, blood thinning, acid reducing, salivary enhancing, and vitamin stimulating life style. Life is good… and then, following a routine follow-up blood test, I'm diagnosed with a mild case of type II diabetes. To many, that would be bad news but for me, knowing it was coming some day, I took it upon myself to make some significant dietary changes – like – divorce Ben and Jerry (both), drop my M&M habit and cut my Dr. Pepper consumption to ZERO... I probably dropped 1,200 calories from my diet over night. The pounds melted off.

As a part of the new routine, Laura and I hit the diabetes web sites to learn about new diet options, blood sugar testing and daily foot inspections. Hey – it's physical attention. One night (during our foot inspection routine), Laura notices an odd spot mark on the bottom of my foot. It's about the size of a large pencil eraser and it's accompanied by two faint streaks, one heading toward the toes, one toward the heel. There's no pain (but I've experienced the "no pain" symptom before and I suffer (mildly) with enduring peripheral neuropathy. A quick check of the web reminds us that a diabetes patient with a black patch of skin is in mortal danger of loosing the foot… it looks bad… It's probably a blood blister… or clogged salivary duct. I can't take time to visit the doctor. Don't they know how important I am?

Off to work for a few days and then, after the prodding from Laura, I decide to show Amy and Kathy Glasgow the foot wound at work. They both immediately responded "you need to have that looked at"… yeah… I'm busy. It doesn't hurt. But I can barely feel my feet at the best of times. After more prodding and phone-number-looking-up, I call and get the appointment.

My primary physician, Dr. Sathar, is a very kind Indian woman that has been working on my blood pressure, cholesterol, weight and overall attitude. I think she likes me (She probably thinks I'm smart). I strip up to the ankle and first show her my big toe's toenail (not why I'm here). It's just a fungus infestation – easily treatable. Then the attention turns to the afflicted foot and it's ugly black spot.

She asks the proverbial questions:

"Does it hurt?"

"How long has it been there?" (I'm thinking, "the foot or the black mark?")

"Did you step on something?"

"What is your favorite color?"

All my answers were quite insightful: "no," "I don't know," "no," and "blue no yellow!" After some picking and prodding to no avail and a few confused looks on her face, she turns to her medical supply drawer, pulls out an alcohol wipe and wipes away the black mark of death.

She chuckled for a very long time. She used to think I was smart.

Chapter 85

My Best Friends: Ben and Jerry

"Message for you Sir."
- Brave, Brave Concorde, Monty Python and the Holy Grail

January 30, 2006

Life continues to be good. We're currently on an airplane heading back to Washington, DC. We just completed a quick weekend visit to my favorite ski resort, Crested Butte, Colorado. OK – life is not that good. We're using my frequent flyer miles and we're in coach. This year the Clower family joined us. The trip got off to a great start with a surprise encounter at the Denver International Airport. Ellen and I had been planning this for about 2 months and my kids (and Laura) had no clue. Their son Brendan walked up to Sarah in the Denver airport Thursday night, handed her a piece of paper with a note on it, and walked away. Sarah was stunned. The weekend was great – super snow and great skiing. The kids picked up right where they left off – Sarah 2 years without a ski pole in her hand - David just last year. 30 minutes in and they were skiing circles around me.

Life with the long-term side effects of cancer treatment is good. The dry mouth and sore neck are the biggies. The neuropathy continues to nag but the numbness in hands, feet and one other important area is just a nuisance. I have calculated the net loss of quality of life due to neuropathy just from the added time to button all the buttons on a dress shirt and it's significant. With an average impact of 23 seconds per day (additional time it takes to button all buttons on a dress shirt), multiplied by 220 days/year over 16.5 years till retirement – the net impact is about 23.2 hours of lost quality of life. I'm determined to put in an insurance claim. At the standard billing rate of $168.75/hour, I'm due $3,913.59. Just above the small claims court limit in the State of California I bet. I'm gonna win one some day.

Dr. Martinez still sees me once a month (our schedules sometimes require a delay). She has told me I can back off to once every 2-3 months at this point. I think I'm about 80% out of the woods. I complain that she only cares about me from the neck up. If I die from something else – she wins! So she sent me off to see a GP. They want to look at everything. I need to get that behind me (sorry for the pun). My weight seems to have stabilized at 170. Diet is a challenge with dry foods still off the menu. I can eat the moist, wonderful Italian breads (given enough butter). Junk foods are still not on the list – but Ben and Jerry are my best friends. Ice cream and help the environment at the same time. It's just like buying organic, free range, chicken broth.

As for the long-term prognoses, I'm basically OK. It's not going to change much from here. I'm not going to eat another pretzel. Butter is my friend. I'm going to die from something else, we're just negotiating when, where, how.

Kids are really growing up. Sarah is thinking about thinking about college. Don't actually mention it to her because she'll stress but she knows she has to think about it some day. I told her she could go anywhere she wants and I'm good with only two constraints: She can NOT live at home and if she goes to Berkeley – she pays.

We're off to school one morning on the last day of the quarter and Sarah is right on the edge. She's worried about her grades and whether we will love her if she ever gets a B. Trying to tell her that my parents gave me up for adoption when I brought home my first A-minus doesn't seem to help. I make her the offer. She knows that Laura and I do not pay for grades. Grades are not important – good grades are their own reward... blah, blah, blah. I tell her, "just this one time, if she can keep it a secret from Mom, I'll give her $10 if she pulls home straight As. I'll give her $50 if she scores a B." She's confused but – she really needs to get a B.

David has all the work ethic of a modern thirteen-year-old boy. If I had had free access to X-BOX 360 I'd be a professional game player – or a bum. Dave is just like me.

Mike

Chapter 86

First Date

"It depends on what the meaning of the word "is" is."
- President, William Jefferson Clinton

I had the privilege of meeting the Honorable Ellen Tauscher, the Livermore Representative to Congress one Saturday afternoon at the Laboratory. Ellen was visiting the lab with Senator Nelson from Florida. Both served on their respective Armed Services Committees and were partnered in pursuit of stable funding for the National Security Complex.

Ellen arrived before the Senator and was welcomed by the Lab senior management in a receiving line like you might see at a wedding reception. Ellen had dealt with the Lab managers before and knew them well (except for me). As she worked her way toward me (at the end of the line), she stopped, exchanged pleasantries, hugs and kisses with each and every person in line (just like a wedding). Ellen got to me, realized she didn't know me and extended her hand for a 1st time handshake. I began to respond and she rethought her strategy – she quickly pulled her hand back as I began to introduce myself and transitioned to the wedding line hug. She whispered in my ear after she kissed me on the cheek "I don't normally kiss on the first date." My response was (predictably) "I do."

Just a few days later, Ellen came back to the Laboratory after winning a major political battle for the benefits of the Laboratory employees. This time, she was to speak in the Lab's main auditorium with the talk televised on the Lab's TV network. She came into a completely packed auditorium and walked the same receiving line of lab managers seated in the front row. I was again at the end of this line. This time, with the Laboratory watching, she walked down the line smiling and shaking hands with the senior managers. She got to me at the end of the line, reached her hand out to shake my hand, pulled it back and gave me a big hug and kiss. I whispered in her ear "I consider this our second date."

She laughed and went on to make a speech that only a politician can. What a great lady.

A few years later, Ellen was diagnosed with esophageal cancer – a very bad hand to be dealt. I'm certain she'll bring all she's got to fight and win that battle.

Ellen Tauscher's got a lot to bring and the world is a better place with Ellen in it!

Chapter 87

The $5,000 Night Stand

"The person that dies with the most frequent flyer miles wins."
- Mike Carter

July 18, 2006

So... Life is good. It's complex, but good. Life deals you the cards and you choose to play them or not. First the health update. After another round of clear throat inspections (still fun), a clear PET scan, clear blood work and another CT scan passed with flying colors, I've decided it's time to prepare to not die from something else – a major turning point in my life. The PET scan was interesting. I walked in, sat in the chair and they opened the safe. The technician pulled out a small lead pig (about the size of your fist) and drew a syringe full of "special sugar." Inserting it into my IV, I asked him what it was? His response ("it's a special sugar") did not surprise me. I was trying to get him to tell me he was going to make me radioactive.

"Radioactive" is a dangerous word in our radio phobic society. We're already radioactive – what's to be afraid of. I asked him if he knew the half-life of the positron emitter (Flourine-18) that he was injecting into my blood stream. He did not... it's 3.5 hours... Oh – how little they know about the positron-electron annihilations they were about ready to create – emitting two coincident 511keV photons – heading in exactly opposite directions (neglecting relativistic effects). Just like Scotty's matter-antimatter reactor on the Enterprise. Physics is good.

With the PET scan clear, CAT scan clear, no recent MRIs, blood work clear, and the throat inspection clear; it is time to actually follow through on the GP recommendations. It's time to check the cholesterol and work to get my blood pressure back down a bit. It had been creeping up to somewhere in the 150/100 range – A macroscopic sign of "doing a good job" at work. I was proud! A cholesterol reading of 278 was not that big a deal two years ago... now – maybe a few less trips to the Rib Eye cut and a little exercise *might be in order. I talked the doctor into cutting me some slack and JUST start me on Cholesterol meds (after promising a divorce from Ben and Jerry). Oh – and prostate clear – The Doctor was gentle...*

The long-term side effects are lessening (but please don't tell anyone). I can't really spit yet and the overall numbness is still a problem weakening my prowess with the women (woman)... But – I'm still a threat. I think I'm just increasingly tolerant of the long-term "norm." Neuropathy is your friend (not!).

All in all – optimism abounds (on the health front).

The work family situation couldn't be more confused. I have recently accepted a fantastic position back at Livermore after four years associated with Homeland Security. The position has lots of words in the title (not a good sign). I'm now the Principal Deputy Associate Director for Nonproliferation, Homeland and International Security (an eight word title not including the "for" and "and"). Gotta work to get the number of words in the title down... That puts me back on the West Coast in my natural habitat.

Laura, Sarah and David will be hanging east for another year... what's not right about this story? I drag them east for my career opportunity and now – I head west. Laura and I decided it was important for Sarah to graduate from TJ – arguably, the best public high school in the country. We'll make it work but – It'll be difficult on our relationship. We just passed the 25 year mark – under celebrated as always. Mom and Aunt Sarah took us all to Morton's steakhouse in Reston. Not the trip to Florence I was thinking about but the company was great. Florence, Kentucky really isn't all that special. Their "David" drives a pickup truck with a shotgun in the back window. The 29 car is his favorite.

Sarah has landed a summer mentorship (research position) in the Chemistry and Material Science Division at LLNL. She's doing a research project on the "nanostructural properties of grain boundary engineered copper." If she were a guy, she'd be dodgeball bait. She has found the world's best mentor (not me this time). Dr. Andrea Hodge – a young Ph.D. material scientist from Columbia (the country) and Northwestern (the university). Sarah has another role model – one who loves life – loves research – loves students. We count our blessings every day. Sarah and David are the ultimate blessings.

I'll settle into a wonderful apartment in Livermore, close to the lab. I'll furnish it with all the amenities a single, married guy needs... computer, TV, bed, microwave, a lamp, and my dog "shithead." My nightstand is a cardboard box – filled with my finest bottles of wine.

Life will be good...

Define good... Good is "life with the ones you love."

Life is good...

Chapter 88

The Portal

"Back off man, I'm a Scientist!"
- Dr. Peter Venkman, Ghostbusters

I take a little bit of pride in knowing my way around Washington, DC. Having lived and worked there for four years and traveled there hundreds of times, I could find my way around traffic, navigate the metro and get into about any federal government office I needed to. My family and colleagues were often surprised (impressed?) that I knew people almost everywhere we went. My family was frequently delayed by my tendency to stop and talk to people I knew – no matter where we were. I knew the ropes (or so I thought).

I had the chance to take a new colleague at work, Kim Budil, around DC and introduce her to my colleagues from across the Government. One morning we were headed to FBI Headquarters to have a discussion with the Director of the Weapons of Mass Destruction (WMD) Directorate. I had spent plenty of time in the Hoover building during my stint in DC trying to build relationships and understand their culture. This sounds easy but if you are not an agent (and don't know their secret handshakes) they can be a tough organization to understand. I had joked with them a few years ago that they were the only Government agency to not have a "send" button on their email system. (This turns out not to be right – there are other agencies without a send button either).

Taking Kim around DC was my chance to show her that I knew the ropes. We entered the new visitor entrance of the Hoover building, went through the metal detectors and got our bags x-rayed. We turned the corner to enter the lobby to get our visitor badges. There was a high-tech portal between the screening area and the badge office. The portal was round with curved glass doors that rotated open and closed for the entrance and exit. As I approached the portal, the entrance door was already rotated open so I stepped in and waited for the door to close and the exit door to rotate open. I stood in the portal for a few seconds and nothing happened. I looked around to see if there was a button to push or something to make the portal work but didn't see anything obvious. With the entrance door still open, I motioned for Kim to step in with me so we could go through together.

We stood very close to each in the portal waiting for something to happen: the entrance door to close and the exit door to open. After a few tens of seconds of waiting and looking around awkwardly, I put my hand on the <u>glass</u> exit door thinking I might push it open... it was already open and had been open the entire time. We just assumed there was a transparent glass door there... We stepped on through (laughing and wondering what the guards looking at the security monitors were thinking about the nerds entering the Hoover Building.)

I really know my way around Washington!

Chapter 89

Hi Mom

"Home is where your Mom hides the popsicles."
- Previously anonymous cancer survivor

October 29, 2006

Today is Laura's Birthday (#48). It's another in a fine line of successes. It's a miracle that she puts up with me. I'm just coming back from a 3-day weekend in Virginia marking not only her 48th but also my 3rd anniversary of the end of my cancer treatments. At the three-year mark, Dr. Martinez only wants to see me about once every three months. My last check-up with her (a few weeks back) was perfect. I'm still all clear as far as she can see. She ordered up another PET scan. At this point, her inspections look mainly for local recurrence. The PET scans look for distant metastasis (liver, bone, lung etc.). Being radioactive for a few hours is a small price to pay for the good feeling you get with a clear PET. At this point, the blood draws, IVs, and scans are just another day at the office. I'm a semi-professional patient. The one-hour nap they insist on after injecting you with the anti-matter emitter is nice. Life is good.

The separation from the family is not fun at all. Sarah is just finishing her application to Stanford University. It's due for consideration for early action on November 1st. Her essays are better than mine so – maybe she has a shot. Stanford is over most everyone's bar and we're an under-the-bar kind of family. By the time I type next, we'll know how much this is going to cost me. Stanford comes in at an estimated $47,500/year. It turns out that all the private schools are almost the same price. It's like wine; if it were cheaper, you would enjoy it less.

Sarah had a great summer at the Lab. Her mentor in Chemistry and Material Science, Andrea Hodge, was absolutely fantastic. She was as encouraging as you can be: encouraging Sarah that she can be a great success AND have fun at the same time (all at her Dad's expense). The "plan" for next summer consists of – using

Dad's money to do something like: go to Europe for a month. "It's my last chance to ever have fun" is the cry from the gallery. Oh – you'll have fun – at the Stanford library. Do Universities even have libraries any more or is it all just on Wikipedia?

Work is a joy. We're in the process of preparing for a contract transition in the management of the laboratory. This is the "end" of the long divorce process between the Department of Energy and the National Labs. It started with Wen Ho Lee at Los Alamos and ends with us worrying about continuity in the retirement system and... lots to worry about. I was part of the contract proposal preparation team (not what I expected when I went to California and left my family in DC but – it's what I got). I'm not as friendly with United Airlines as I would like but I am making it home enough to remember the garage door code and not have the kids call 911 when they see me. Lucky for me, I still buy them drinks at Starbucks.

Life is good. God willing, my PET scan will be clear and I'll be proof reading this in a few weeks. I'm on a mission to get this book done and "published." My audience is calling... it's a lonely voice but one I recognize... "Hi Mom."

Love to all, Mike

Chapter 90

Second Opinions

"Scientists should be on tap, but not on top."
- Sir Winston Churchill

In May of 2008, I had the opportunity to participate in a visit to the Laboratory by General Jeff Smith. General Smith was assigned to the National Security Council at the time and was asked by Steven Hadley, the then National Security Advisor to President Bush, to get an answer to the often-asked question: Why do we have two nuclear weapons laboratories (Los Alamos and Lawrence Livermore)? Well, at Livermore, we know that question well. It really means: Why do we have Livermore Lab – the "second laboratory?" Our colleagues/competitors at Los Alamos hear the same question quite differently: "Why would anyone ever need more than our expertise? The rivalry between the lab goes back to the early 1950s when the "joke" was: "The Russians are the competition, Los Alamos is the enemy."

We had endured this line of questioning before (never with my participation). My boss was on travel for the day and I got to play the role of the Principal Associate Director for Global Security (the National Security Programs at LLNL that are not directly associated with the maintenance of the Nation's nuclear weapons stockpile.) It was a wonderful day starting with a tour of the nuclear weapons vault at LLNL. The vault is a very secure room where we display models showing the details of the nation's nuclear weapons (without special nuclear material or real high explosives). The models are used as props to tell the story of LLNL's contributions over the years to the safe, secure, reliable, high-performance stockpile of today. There are many compelling stories of LLNL's contributions often challenging the conventional wisdom and the thinking of the "First Laboratory": Los Alamos. Many of the stories have fascinating physics and engineering details behind them – stories easy for us to tell. Challenges in materials, super computing and nuclear physics that have led to the modern stockpile are the things we take the most pride in. They are also the most challenging to talk about: especially to a history major.

General Smith was a bright, respectful one-star general but the story he was getting was not for him. He asked that the hour at the end of day be reserved for the final discussion on "why we have two labs?" That final discussion began the only way we know how to do it: repeating the interesting, technically complex challenges that were the basis of the modern stockpile – many benefiting significantly from the peer review and competition of ideas between the labs. There were the grand challenges about certification of the stockpile without nuclear testing, utilizing the world's largest super computers and an emerging method called Quantitative Measures of Uncertainty (QMU), and plutonium aging, and blah, blah, blah, yada, yada, yada. All these are great stories but they were not capturing the history major. I decided to wait for a pause and inject a different line of reasoning about the need for two, technically capable, world-class laboratories working the hard, critically important problems and getting to the best answer.

That pause came and I somewhat reluctantly began with: "I'd like to tell a quick story that makes the point a different way."

The Lab director, George Miller, looked at me with that "I wonder where the hell this is going" look on his face.

"Five years ago, I was faced with a personal life and death situation. I had been diagnosed with stage IV throat cancer and the statistics told me I had about a 20% chance of living another five years." I was certain he had noticed the gruesome scar on the side of my neck (actually most people claim they miss it completely) or the bottle of water I carry around with me everywhere I go, including the nuclear weapons vault – where no water has gone before. Both are telltale signs of a throat cancer survivor.

"My healthcare provider was (and still is) Kaiser Permanente. Kaiser is the largest HMO in California and has a reputation of being the low-cost (efficient) provider with a set of good (but maybe not the greatest) physicians. Kaiser was known for quickly diagnosing your condition and getting you in a treatment program and completing the treatment – quickly. I had been told by many people how important it was to be absolutely sure the diagnosis was correct before starting the treatment. I was bound and determined to get a second opinion. My life was at stake."

I could see the lab's most senior management giving me some rope on this story but it had better be good and quick. Undeterred, I continued. "I went to Kaiser and told them I needed a second opinion. They suggested that I visit another Doctor (with an office right next door to my head and neck surgeon). I wouldn't have to have any new tests run. I wouldn't have to take my files with me. He could just call up my case on the computer and render me a second opinion. We could do this the next day. It would be very quick, very efficient and very inexpensive. I told them: This was not a second opinion, this was a first opinion a second time." I could see the analog to the weapons program as clear as day but I had never told this story before (and thus no one had ever heard it). I was climbing out on my limb. I kept sawing.

"Kaiser then suggested that I visit a Kaiser facility in Oakland where I could talk to a head and neck physician (also in the Kaiser system). Again, I wouldn't have to have any more tests run. I wouldn't have to take my files. The Doctor could just call my file up on his computer and render a second opinion. They again made the case about how easy that would be for me. And again – how quick and efficient (and inexpensive) this would be. I told them this was a little bit better but given that the physician was hired into the Kaiser system and was likely employing the same basic practices of a Kaiser physician – concerned about his patients but also "bought into" the Kaiser treatment model – I needed an opinion from "outside" their system. I wanted to go to Stanford's head and neck department." This story was getting a bit long so, I needed to get to the point.

"Kaiser then told me how complex that would be. Stanford would order up new tests. I would have to take my file (including the films of the CAT scans and MRIs) and new slides of my tumor would have to be cut, mounted and shipped to Stanford. All these things would be expensive and time consuming. They would do it but they would not pay for it. I told them it was my life on the line and I didn't care how expensive it was or who was paying for it. I wanted to have Stanford render an opinion to confirm that the path I was about to embark on, with my life in the balance, was in fact the best path."

"I proceeded to go to Stanford with my file and get that second, independent opinion from world-class physicians knowing that my treatment would be done by Kaiser. I did have to pay "a lot of money" (not really) for access to this expertise. In the end, the second opinion was different enough to change my treatment course. Maybe that change was small but it also made me more confident that the more aggressive treatment path that I chose was the treatment that gave me the best prognosis – not just the most efficient and inexpensive path. I started the treatment more confident that I was on the best path. That was worth the money. That's what I call a "second opinion.""

"Nuclear weapons are a similar story. The issues in the stockpile are critically important that the nation get them right. This often requires a top notch, second opinion on even the seemingly most insignificant issues. In cancer diagnosis and the nuclear stockpile, there is too much at stake to allow too much "efficiency" to get in the way of getting the right answer. Two independent, technically capable laboratories provide that second opinion."

General Smith replied, "I'm not sure I understand plutonium aging but I get that story." I had made the point and the director didn't fire me. Who says cancer can't be a good thing?

Chapter 91

National Nothing Day

"It's always something. If it ain't one thing, it's another."
- Roseanne Roseannadana

March 25, 2007

So... today is a special day. Special in that there is nothing special today. This is rare in the days of "National Arbor day," "President's day," and "National vasectomy day." Maybe this should be "National Nothing day." It's likely someone's birthday, anniversary or whatever but not anything I know about and I'm not looking. Statistically, the only day less likely to have nothing happening (assuming all events happen randomly) is February 29th. 25% as likely than March 25th – but comes around 25% less often. You do the math.

So much good is going on in our lives. We're on track to get back together! We've purchased a house in California (one that Laura has yet to see except in digital pictures). We have sold our house in Virginia! It's a miracle of miracles – in a slow market. The house had two offers in two days. The real estate agent says it looked good. Sarah has college offers rolling in. UC Santa Barbara is the first to show. Following closely with offers were UC Davis, University of Virginia, and Cal Tech.

Holding up the show are Stanford, Harvey Mudd, UC San Diego, and Duke. I can't see her with blue and white stripes on her face. We're planning a Southern California college tour with stops at the beach in Santa Barbara and La Jolla (UCSD) on the docket. Spring break will be a dud for David but we'll make it work somehow. Maybe we'll play some Frisbee golf at each campus or soap the fountains. All acceptances are expected by the end of the week (April 1) and – she must decide by May 1. Good time to be in another state. Turn down Cal Tech for???? She might. It's supposed to be her decision, not mine.

This has been an interesting health care time. Trips to the doctor now are centered on my blood pressure... I think it's high... they don't. No medications until I can get my pressure up a bit. Exercise (if you call it that) and diet are not working for me. I'll try to sit and watch more TV, use more salt, or just spend more time at work.

I'm rapidly approaching the April 2 anniversary of my diagnosis. Almost four years has passed and what do I have to show for it?: ninety pages of italicized text and a new lease on life. I've decided to become obsessive compulsive again. My obsessions will be – no wasting time, concentrate on positive engagement with everyone around me, exercise 210 minutes per week, and keep up with the Clowers. I'm sure that last one violates some commandment, law, or zoning restriction. Make them come get me.

Mike

Chapter 92

Why?

"*The lord is subtle, but malicious he is not.*"
  - Albert Einstein

Everybody has a "why?" Why do people write cancer books? Lance Armstrong's why was: to show survival against all odds, to win even if he had to break the rules, to remain determined in the face of adversity, renewed focus on the important things in life (he divorced his wife after surviving cancer – maybe he's not any more perfect than the next guy). Focus and determination are powerful tools in the fight against adversity. Cancer is an iconic adversary that will directly afflict 20-50% of people in their lifetimes. Almost no one can relate to Lance as a bike rider but almost half of us can relate to Lance as a cancer victim. Lance is a role model for cancer patients in need of focus and determination. No – Lance is THE role model for focus and determination. In other areas, Lance may not be the place to look.

Lots of people *appear* to have a "why." King Arthur had a "why": "The lady of the lake, her arm clad in the pure simmering Semite, held aloft from the bosom of the water, Excalibur! That's why I'm your King!" ("Strange women lying in ponds distributing swords is no basis for a system of government. Supreme executive power is derived from a mandate from the masses, not from some farcical aquatic ceremony.") You get the point. President Kennedy *did* have a "why?" - made clear to us all by the end results: the Cuban missile crisis and the man on the moon. A single gunman in Dallas took him from us but his "why" has endured. His "why?" is cemented in history. My "why?" is still in the formative stages.

Maybe this book is my "Why?" Maybe my "why" is showing others that challenge and adversity can be met head on and conquered - with humor. Maybe I don't need bike races, or vision to place man on the moon, or "moistened binks lobbing scimitars at me." Or maybe some things are just not meant to be known.

Maybe there is a simple theory. Maybe I have to define my own purpose! My own "why?" Maybe I shouldn't wait for a divine strike or a vision of the Virgin Mary in my ice cube tray. Maybe it's there in front of me, my own special purpose.

It's so empowering, so uplifting, and so special. And – I can change it! Whenever, wherever, whyever, as often as, I want. It can be plural. It probably shouldn't be too plural if it's "special." "Special purposes" might be only limited to only a few special purpi per person (purpi is the scientific plural of purpose). It is mine! It's what makes me good and what makes me evil. It's what makes me human. It's what makes me special.

Given this theory, one might ask, what is my special purpose? I have no idea! But it's mine. I've been thinking about adopting Navin R. Johnson's but it's already taken.

A few guiding principles: trustworthy, loyal, helpful, friendly, courteous, kind, obedient, cheerful, thrifty, brave, clean and reverent. Wait – that's my Eagle Scout stuff. Actually, the Boy Scout stuff captures the core values pretty well: integrity, honesty, bravery, and smelling nice. But I point out that it misses some others: humor, resiliency, resistance, adaptiveness, persistence, creativity, leadership, and teamwork. There should be a Viola Joke merit badge. I know there is no Persistence merit badge but it is the most important trait to get a weak swimmer through the lifesaving merit badge, set the high score on the Fireball pinball machine, lead an experimental campaign in Siberia, or deal with the hiccups in the throws of chemotherapy-induced depression.

Persistence should not be mistaken for "going it alone." "Going it alone" is almost always the second best choice. I believe in a much better idea: use "the others." Making others more effective and developing common vision and a sense of purpose is much more powerful. Leadership can't solve everything but when change is needed, leadership brings together the forces required to evolve. Maybe that's my special purpose. Maybe that's my "why?"

Maybe my purpose is to bring purpose (or purpi) to others. With that in mind, I tell my cancer story. I did not ask for this story. This story unfolded upon me. The struggle to survive is fought in many ways. The fight is one of persistence and, more importantly, a fight with others on my side. I never once fought alone and I always fought with humor. Alone, there is likely no success and there is certainly no humor. With humor, I was never alone. With others, I was never without humor.

Whether we know it or not, we all live on the edge. I try to not just look around; I try, at least once in a while, to look over the edge.

I try to laugh and smile. Both are contagious. Maybe not as contagious as H5N1 or a yawn, but a smile is longer lasting. Then again, nothing is as contagious as a yawn.

Chapter 93

Best Suit, Inside Pocket

"I never saw a pessimistic General win a battle."
- General Dwight D. Eisenhower

May 30, 2007

It's my birthday, my anniversary, and my four-year survival mark (self proclaimed date)... In case you haven't realized, this story does not have an ending. This might be a disappointment for those making the movie or those that read the end of the book before the beginning (I look in the mirror as I type). This story would be much worse (and written by someone else) if the cancer had returned. It's always a threat and I must admit there are times when I think about the cancer returning. I'll get a sore throat or "feel a lump" and the fear creeps closer. I try to keep it to the doctors and myself. There is no sense in scaring anyone else. I expect this won't change. It's part of being vigilant. So far – I'm clear – and vigilant – and scared.

On the positive side, this story would be so much better if it ended with me winning the Nobel Prize or the Escape from Alcatraz or a Tour d' France title. It would be better if you were witness to me paying off my bet with my friend August Droege. August and I have a bet on who will die first. If I win, the pay off ($20 bill) is in the breast pocket of my best suit. She'll have to reach in for it. Watch for an act of distraction at my funeral – she's tricky. If she wins, I'm reaching in for my payout wherever she might be hiding that bill. But no. It's more like real life where endings are anti-climatic. I'm not in the running for the Nobel Prize (Physics or Peace). I'm not training for a marathon or bike race or other test of endurance. I'm trying to get this book done and I'm trying to learn how to spit. If you can't spit, you can't run a marathon – it's a rule. I do have a $20 bill in my suit pocket – just in case.

I'm at the four-year mark planning the combined five-year cancer-free anniversary, 50th birthday and 27th anniversary party. This book comes with an invitation (BYOBS – Bring Your Own Booze

245

and Story (or Bring Your Own BS)). It also comes with hope. Hope for a great future. There is so much to do but unfortunately, more than we all can do in a lifetime. This is especially true if you include the things worth doing more than once.

Much has been accomplished. The family is almost back together – in California. Sarah has accepted the offer from the University of Virginia. Caltech came in third! They are shattered. My mountaineering prowess has been reestablished by multiple returns to Yosemite including a recent, nearly failed trek to the Diving Board (my favorite place in the world – with one of my favorite people – John Scarafiotti). My next plan – get my brother and son up there. After that – I will have one less thing to live for. I still have Danica Patrick and Kate Austin to root for. Danica has not won Indy yet and Kate is still on that damn Lost Island. I have hope for both of them. In the mean time, Laura keeps me away from Speedway, Indiana and obscure islands in the South Pacific (like the west coast of Oahu).

There is much to reflect on and learn from. I remember my Dad. His early passing at age 67 deprived my children of the greatest grandfather the world has ever known. We still cherish the ornaments he painted with the kids in the basement. He could read to the kids and snore in the same sitting. We remember fondly how he would cut a slice of apple with his pocketknife, stab the slice with the tip of the knife blade and extend the skewered apple toward the innocent four year old in his unique attempt to share. Dad continues to be my role model in supporting my children. He was always proud and unwavering in his commitment. He provided me with much-needed "top cover" to the end... May I live to such a high standard.

My struggles with long-lasting side effects have been reduced to – sore neck, dry mouth, trouble swallowing, neuropathy, the occasional Marcia, Marcia, Marcia, and a great case of such small things to complain about. As I like to say, my sick cards are running out. Finally, after four years, conversations do not begin with, get interrupted by, or end with discussions about cancer. The doctors don't want to see me as much anymore. People don't see *me as a cancer survivor first anymore. To me that means – I am a survivor. It's no longer about the cancer or the struggle to survive. I've survived. It's now about fighting the next thing that might kill me. Whatever that is. Until that emerges, it's about doing something to make the world a better place? What am I doing to make the people around me great? How to care for my family? It's finally about the enduring things that are important to me. It's now about life.*

Life is good... very good...

Mike

Chapter 94

Is Somebody Watching?

"Your theory is crazy, but it's not crazy enough to be true."
- Niels Bohr

We've been known to enjoy a weekend away at Sea Ranch, a very nice "community" just up the Northern California coast from San Francisco. Sea Ranch is a wonderfully peaceful place. It's a few hundred houses along about twenty miles of coastline with wonderful hiking trails along the bluffs. It's a great place to rent a house for the weekend and get away from it all. We typically will rent a house with the Clower family and the eight of us (plus hangers-on) will spend a few days resting, eating, hiking, eating, tide pooling, eating, and reflecting on the world.

On one particular visit, the skies on Friday night were unusually clear along the coast. One could see the Milky Way as clear as ever from the balcony of the house overlooking the Pacific Ocean. Ellen Tarwater-Clower and I decided to venture out, getting even further away from the already sparse lights, and check out the heavens. Ellen had just returned from a church group visit to Palestine where she had seen first hand both sides of the epic, never-ending struggle. Her church group had organized a trip to a small Palestinian community that was experimenting with multi-cultural education with their young people. This is a surefire formula for success in a region of the world desperate for good ideas. Ellen had come back more firmly convinced than ever that the world could be a better place.

On our walk that night we talked about all the good (and evil) in the world. We talked about religion – her faith and my convictions: that the world is "governed" by the laws of nature – gravity and quantum mechanics. It's actually ruled by relativistic quantum mechanics to be exact (pending the outcome of the grand unified field theory), although, the correction terms are not very important to most macroscopic phenomena. Ellen and I come down on the same side of almost everything except my "threat status" and religion. We agreed to the same purposes in life but agreed to pursue them in different ways (as we always do). It was a great talk on a memorable evening with an absolutely awesome lady.

The next day, Ellen and I went for a walk along the coast. It was low tide so we ventured down to the waters' edge to do a little tide pooling (remember – the northern California coast is not a beach, it is rocky bluffs with cold water, and vicious, unpredictable wave action). I am scared to death of the ocean. Its power and unpredictable nature is intimidating like no other force (except maybe a girl). We're down at the edge of the waves, looking at the animal life in the tide pools (Ellen is a good bit closer to the waters' edge than I – and much less afraid). Out of nowhere (just like they always do) came a rogue wave. It crashed into the rocks and a huge wall of water was launched into the air. This rogue column of saltwater (obeying all the laws of physics that apply to columns of saltwater) leapt toward the heavens as though it had a mind of its own, clearing Ellen, and coming back to earth drenching me. Ellen looked up at me smiling (or maybe laughing) and calmly remarked, "He was listening last night."

The wise man would leave it at that, maybe reflect a little, probably not retell the story too much and certainly not brag about the attention drenched upon him. I'm not frequently referred to as "wise."

A few months later, a friend from Washington, Huban Gowadia, made her way to California and we took a trip to Yosemite Valley. It was one of those spectacular days in the most beautiful valley on earth. It had snowed between six and twelve inches the night before and the valley was absolutely beautiful. As we hiked, I retold the story of the rogue wave and Ellen's interpretation of the event. Huban laughed and chalked it up to another failed opportunity for Mike to understand the world beyond relativistic quantum physics.

As we hiked down from Vernal Falls through the slowly melting snow, Huban asked me if I still liked Evangeline Lilly (my favorite TV actress from the show *Lost*). I reminded her that "I was a guy, with a pulse, who could fog a mirror and increase the entropy in the universe and, as such, of course I like boobs." It wasn't a half second from the time the word "boobs" came out of my mouth until I was hit right on the top of the head by a large chuck of snow falling from the tree above the trail. The timing was such that the snowball left the tree branch after the thought was formed in my mind but BEFORE the word "boobs" was uttered. It was like someone knew what I was thinking and maybe thought it is was inappropriate.

Huban's immediate response (having just heard the story about the rogue wave): "God 2, Mike 0."

More likely, the square of the product of the two wave functions was non-zero. The relativistic terms can generally be neglected.

Chapter 95

One hell of a day

*"I am an optimist.
It does not seem too much use being anything else."*
- Sir Winston Churchill

May 30, 2008

May was a very challenging month. As I had promised in May of 2003, I was bound and determined to have a victory celebration on Friday, May 30. The confluence of events was too good to pass up. My 50th birthday, our 27th wedding anniversary, and my self-proclaimed 5-year cancer survival point all coincided on the same day. And Kate had finally made it off the island. The word was out and we were poised to have a party. The invitations were on the street. We had invited the Vice President (Dick Cheney), Rachel Ray, Kate Austin (Evangeline Lilly), and 200 of my closest friends from all over the country to our home for dinner. Exactly what we were thinking was not clear. We thought Cheney might not make it, Rachel had yet to respond, and it's not clear what year Kate Austin was living in at the time but I was sure she was coming.

Life does have a way of throwing curve balls. The week before the party, my wife was given notice of her layoff from the laboratory after 26 years of service. The laboratory was undergoing significant downsizing as the Government's commitment to the nuclear weapons program was being "right-sized." The Friday before our party was one of the roughest days of our lives. Laura had been let go from the laboratory – her employer for more than 20 years. Invited to our celebration were Laura's boss, his boss, and his boss's boss. There were many pieces of advise from our friends: Cancel, move the venue, run and hide. One evening, a few days before the party, Laura stood up to our friends and said "No! We're hosting the damn party!" We were bound and determined to celebrate a 5-year journey – in the face of a new challenge.

Celebrate we did. Who would have thought you could host a sit down dinner (served buffet style) for 150 people in your home? An old friend from my days in the Nuclear Testing program, Carl Bruns, was the primary chef. He's quite experienced at grilling chicken and tri-tip in 55-gallon drums in the back yard. Add wine, beer, beans, salad, rolls, brownies, and ice cream and you have a party. The 120 real wine glasses from Costco (not the plastic crap) were the service plan for the 40+ bottles of wine (all Robert Parker 90+ points) that we plowed through. It was an absolutely wonderful way to express my thanks for the support of my family and friends.

I had the chance of a lifetime to give a profound speech to the people I cared most about. I wish I knew what I said. It was unrehearsed and I'm sure it was quite profound. Some of the kids gave me the two finger ("we've heard this before") sign and laughed out loud. Laura even said a few words in a rare "public" speaking moment. I can only imagine the courage it took to stand in front of her family, friends, and former work colleagues and speak from the heart. I can't remember a single word she used but I know exactly what she said.

As John Scarafiotti reminded me that night, "You're one lucky guy." Maybe. Maybe I'm fortunate. Or maybe I hang around lucky people. Joe Ronchetto called me "peckerhead" that night and Ellen Tarwater-Clower reminded me that I'm still "not a threat." My wife told me, silently, how much she loved me.

That night I went to bed, exhausted and fulfilled; challenged and blessed; full of love and loved. I was confident that life is good and there is much more life ahead of me.

*In closing, there are a few things I'm stuck with:
dry salivary glands,
a "beautiful" neck scar,
neuropathy,
great friends,
the greatest family,
an ever-improving wine collection,
a bucket list that grows instead of shrinks,
a $20 bill in the breast pocket of my best suit,
and eternal optimism.*

Save room in the coffin for my wine collection.

I might not be a threat but I am one lucky guy!

Thanks

"It's hard to beat a person who never gives up."
- Babe Ruth

I'd like to thank my friends and family for the encouragement to battle cancer and complete this book. Many of them were right there with me in 2003 as I worked my way through the uncertainty of stage IV cancer diagnosis and treatment. Not one of them sold me short (that I know of)!

The thanks to my wife cannot be put into words (or gifts). I could try but I would fail. She has not read this book and you now know why.

I owe much of my early educations on cancer to Christine Hartmann. She jumped to my rescue at that critical "what is happening?" stage and never gave up hope!

Special thanks to my daughter Sarah whose guidance protected me and, more importantly, those I wrote about. Her good judgment and editing skills were critical to getting this done. My son David has always been there for me through good and bad. My mother is a saint. My brother is the best!

Please remember those who have fought and are no longer with us. My Dad died much too early and missed so much. He would be so proud of his four grandchildren.

Thanks to all of you who helped edit and motivate this book. Dr. Huban Gowadia provided much encouragement and editorial comment along the way. She would prefer to remain anonymous but that is not possible.

I am ever indebted to Bob Sadler, a fellow cancer survivor, photographer and friend who gave critical advice and encouragement in the early stages of the preparation of this book. Bob is a true gem who continues to motivate me every day.

Sandy Jackson gets special mention as the final motivator to get this out!

Special thanks to Lance Armstrong for helping me reach one of my goals: Winning the same number of Tour d' France races as you have. It's always good to have help for the most challenging of life's goals. I have always believed it is NOT ok to lie and cheat if you think you might get away with it.

Did I mention my Doctors? I trusted them and they delivered.

Thanks again to my friends and family! Without you this wouldn't have been worth it.

About the Author:

Michael Carter lives in Livermore, California and has worked at Lawrence Livermore National Laboratory since 1981. In 2003, while on assignment in Washington, DC working to help establish the Department of Homeland Security, he was diagnosed with Stage IV throat cancer. During his "vacation" he chronicled his journey through cancer treatment in a weekly series of letters to his friends and family. Mike is married with two grown children: Sarah and David.

This is Mike's first book.

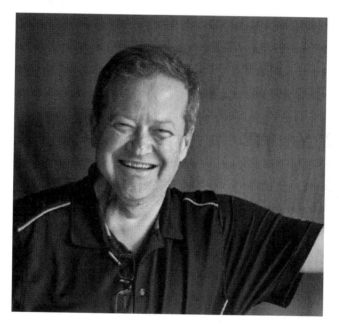

Photo by the <u>great</u> Jamie Douglas

Mike is an avid photographer.

Follow him at <u>www.mikecarterphotograph.com</u>

Mike is a cancer survivor.

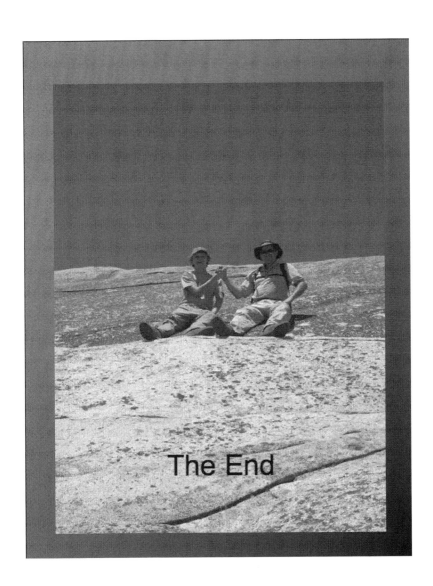

Made in the USA
San Bernardino, CA
03 October 2015